Oxford Case
Histories in
Rheumatology

Oxford Case Histories
Series Editors
Sarah Pendlebury and Peter Rothwell

Published:
Neurological Case Histories (Sarah Pendlebury, Philip Anslow, and Peter Rothwell)

Oxford Case Histories in Cardiology (Rajkumar Rajendram, Javed Ehtisham, and Colin Forfar)

Oxford Case Histories in Gastroenterology and Hepatology (Alissa Walsh, Otto Buchel, Jane Collier, and Simon Travis)

Oxford Case Histories in Respiratory Medicine (John Stradling, Andrew Stanton, Anabell Nickol, Helen Davies, and Najib Rahman)

Oxford Case Histories in Rheumatology (Joel David, Anne Miller, Anushka Soni, and Lyn Williamson)

Forthcoming:
Oxford Case Histories in Neurosurgery (Harutomo Hasegawa, Matthew Crocker, and Pawanjit Singh Minhas)

Oxford Case Histories in TIA and Stroke (Sarah Pendlebury, Ursula Schulz, Aneil Malhotra, and Peter Rothwell)

Oxford Case Histories in Rheumatology

Joel David
Consultant Rheumatologist and Lead Physician,
Nuffield Orthopaedic Centre,
Oxford, UK

Anne Miller
Associate Specialist in Rheumatology,
Nuffield Orthopaedic Centre,
Oxford, UK

Anushka Soni
Clinical Lecturer in Rheumatology,
University of Oxford,
Oxford, UK

Lyn Williamson
Consultant Rheumatologist,
Great Western Hospital,
Swindon, UK

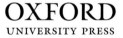

OXFORD
UNIVERSITY PRESS

OXFORD

UNIVERSITY PRESS

Great Clarendon Street, Oxford ox2 6DP

Oxford University Press is a department of the University of Oxford.
It furthers the University's objective of excellence in research, scholarship,
and education by publishing worldwide in

Oxford New York

Auckland Cape Town Dar es Salaam Hong Kong Karachi
Kuala Lumpur Madrid Melbourne Mexico City Nairobi
New Delhi Shanghai Taipei Toronto

With offices in

Argentina Austria Brazil Chile Czech Republic France Greece
Guatemala Hungary Italy Japan Poland Portugal Singapore
South Korea Switzerland Thailand Turkey Ukraine Vietnam

Oxford is a registered trade mark of Oxford University Press
in the UK and in certain other countries

Published in the United States
by Oxford University Press Inc., New York

British Library Cataloguing in Publication Data
Data available

Library of Congress Cataloguing in Publication Data
Library of Congress Control Number: 2011939859

Typeset in Minion by Cenveo, Bangalore, India
Printed in Great Britain
on acid-free paper by
CPI Group (UK) Ltd, Croydon, CR0 4YY

ISBN 978–0–19–958750–6

10 9 8 7 6 5 4 3 2 1

A note from the series editors

Case histories have always had an important role in medical education, but most published material has been directed at undergraduates or residents. The Oxford Case Histories series aims to provide more complex case-based learning for clinicians in specialist training and consultants, with a view to aiding preparation for entry- and exit-level specialty examinations or revalidation.

Each case book follows the same format with approximately 50 cases, each comprising a brief clinical history and investigations, followed by questions on differential diagnosis and management, and detailed answers with discussion.

All cases are peer-reviewed by Oxford consultants in the relevant specialty. At the end of each book, cases are listed by mode of presentation, aetiology, and diagnosis. We are grateful to our colleagues in the various medical specialties for their enthusiasm and hard work in making the series possible.

Sarah Pendlebury and Peter Rothwell

From reviews of other books in the series:

Neurological Case Histories
'...contains 51 cases that cover the spectrum of acute neurology and the neurology of general medicine—this breadth makes the volume unique and provides a formidable challenge... it is a heavy-duty diagnostic series of cases, and readers have to work hard, to recognise the diagnosis and answer the questions that are posed for each case... I recommend this excellent volume highly...'
Lancet Neurology

'This short and well-written text is...designed to enhance the reader's diagnostic ability and clinical understanding...A well-documented and practical book.'
European Journal of Neurology

Oxford Case Histories in Gastroenterology and Hepatology
'...a fascinating insight in to clinical gastroenterology, an excellent and enjoyable read and an education for all levels of gastroenterologist from ST1 to consultant.'
Gut

Preface

This book contains a series of case histories that the authors have encountered in the Oxford region. The purpose of the cases is to provide trainees, and indeed all practitioners in rheumatology, with clinical scenarios and an evidenced approach to answering questions raised by the cases. It is hoped that the book will be useful for training as well as in preparation for exit examinations. The book may also be helpful for rheumatologists in their re-validation. General medical trainees might find it useful in preparation for MRCP and PACES.

Many of the cases require clinical judgement in the approach to the management decisions and questions. The authors have expressed their views and hope that you generally agree! The cases cover inflammatory joint and connective tissue disease, paediatric rheumatology, sports and exercise medicine, and metabolic bone disease. Some of the cases include acute presentations and others are more chronic musculoskeletal and mechanical problems where there are dilemmas in clinical practice.

The authors have used the format of case reports, with detailed discussions of differential diagnosis and management, for three reasons. First, one of the best ways to learn advanced clinical medicine is through the analysis of individual cases. In almost all areas of medicine it is extremely difficult to illustrate the practical process of diagnosis within the format of a traditional textbook. Secondly, it is simply more interesting to consider real cases than to read a text. This allows a clinician to reflect on their own differential diagnosis and treatment. Finally, there is a lack of case series that stretch the abilities of experienced clinicians and specialists: most are aimed at medical students or young doctors doing early postgraduate exams. It is for this reason that the cases and questions are sometimes challenging, although many are simple since the aim is to educate. Wherever possible radiology and clinical pictures have been included.

The authors would like to thank their colleagues, including those allied to medicine, for contributing cases and providing illustrations or administrative support. The clinicians who contributed cases are listed in the Acknowledgements.

We hope you enjoy the book!

Joel David
Anne Miller
Anushka Soni
Lyn Williamson

Acknowledgements

Dr Kuljeet Bhamra

Miss Jane Flynn

Dr Lawrence John

Dr Maria Juarez

Dr Sarah Keidel

Ms Fiona Kinnear

Dr Lucy Mackillop

Dr Kulveer Mankia

Dr Brendan McDonald

Dr Ishita Patel

Dr Elizabeth Price

Dr Nick Ridley

Dr Joanna Robson

Dr Shilpa Selvan

Dr Bill Smith

Dr Anisha Sodha

Dr Ravi Suppiah

Dr Rosemary Waller

Dr Thamindu Wedatilake

Dr Luke Williamson

Contents

Abbreviations

AAS	atlanto-axial subluxation	CTX	carboxy-terminal collagen crosslinks
ABPI	ankle–brachial pressure index	CXR	chest X-ray
ACCP	anticitrullinated C-peptide (also referred to as ACPA)	DAS	Disease Activity Score
ACE	angiotensin-converting enzyme	DEXA	dual-energy X-ray absorptiometry
aCL	anticardiolipin antibody	DILS	diffuse infiltrative lymphocytosis syndrome
ALP	alkaline phosphatase		
ANA	antinuclear antibody	DISH	diffuse idiopathic skeletal hyperostosis
ANCA	antineutrophil cytoplasmic antibody		
		DMARD	disease-modifying anti-rheumatic drug
AND	adverse neural dynamics		
APS	antiphospholipid syndrome	EBV	Epstein–Barr virus
APTT	activated partial thromboplastin time	ECG	electrocardiogram
		EF	eosinophilic fasciitis
AS	ankylosing spondylitis	EIA	enzyme immunoassay
ASOT	antistreptolysin-O titre	ELISA	enzyme-linked immunosorbent assay
AST	aspartate transaminase		
BASDAI	Bath Ankylosing Spondylitis Disease Activity Index	EMG	electromyography
		ENA	extractable nuclear antigen
BD	Behçet's disease	ESR	erythrocyte sedimentation rate
BMD	bone mineral density	EULAR	European League Against Rheumatism
BMI	body mass index		
BSR	British Society for Rheumatology	FBC	full blood count
CK	creatine kinase	FMF	familial Mediterranean fever
CMV	cytomegalovirus	FSH	follicle-stimulating hormone
CNSV	central nervous system vasculitic	GACNS	granulomatous angiitis of the central nervous system
COX-2	cyclo-oxgenase-2	GCA	giant cell arteritis
CPK	creatine phosphokinase	GFR	glomerular filtration rate
CREST	calcinosis, Raynaud's, (o)esphageal involvement, sclerodactyly, telangiectasia	GGT	gamma glutamyl transferase
		GH	growth hormone
		GPA	granulomatosis with polyangiitis (also known as Wegener's granulomatosis (WG))
CRMO	chronic relapsing multifocal osteomyelitis		
CRP	C-reactive protein	HA	haemophiliac arthropathy
CRPS	complex regional pain syndrome	Hb	haemoglobin
CSF	cerebrospinal fluid	HLA	human leucocyte antigen
CSS	Churg–Strauss syndrome	hpf	high-power field
CT	computed tomography		

IBD	inflammatory bowel disease	PFJ	patello-femoral joint
IGF-1	insulin-like growth factor 1	PFPS	patello-femoral pain syndrome
INR	international normalized ratio	PMR	polymyalgia rheumatica
IP	interphalangeal	PT	prothrombin time
IRIS	immune reconstitution inflammatory syndrome	PTH	parathyroid hormone
		PTT	partial thromboplastin time
JIA	juvenile idiopathic arthritis	PUK	peripheral ulcerative keratitis
LA	lupus anticoagulant	PUO	pyrexia of unknown origin
LDH	lactate dehydrogenase	RA	rheumatoid arthritis
LFT	liver function test	RBC	red blood cell
LH	luteinizing hormone	RCVS	reversible cerebral vasoconstrictive syndrome
MAGIC	mouth and genital ulcers with inflamed cartilage		
		RF	rheumatoid factor
MAS	macrophage activation syndrome	RP	relapsing polychondritis
		SAP	serum amyloid protein
MCP	metacarpophalangeal	SAPHO	synovitis, acne, pustulosis, hyperostosis, and osteitis
MCV	mean cell volume		
MEN-I	multiple endocrine neoplasia I	SD	standard deviation
MHC	major histocompatibility complex	SHBG	sex-hormone-binding globulin
		SLE	systemic lupus erythematosus
MPA	microscopic polyangiitis	SOJIA	systemic-onset juvenile idiopathic arthritis
MRA	magnetic resonance angiography		
		STIR	short T_1 inversion recovery
MRI	magnetic resonance imaging	TakA	Takayasu's arteritis
MSCRAMM	microbial surface components recognizing adhesive matrix molecules	TENS	transcutaneous electrical nerve stimulation
		TFT	thyroid function test
MTSS	medial tibial stress syndrome	TGF-β	transforming growth factor-β
NICE	National Institute of Clinical Excellence	TNF	tumour necrosis factor
		TPHA	*Treponema pallidum* haemagglutination test
NOF	neck of the femur		
NSAID	non-steroidal anti-inflammatory drug	TSH	thyroid-stimulating hormone
		U&E	urea and electrolytes
NSIP	non-specific interstitial pneumonia	VAS	Visual Analogue Score
		VDRL	Venereal Disease Research Laboratory
NTX	cross-linked N-telopeptides of type 1 collagen		
		VMO	vastus medialis obliterans
NYHA	New York Heart Association	VS	ventral subluxation
OA	osteoarthritis	VTE	venous thromboembolism
OI	osteogenesis imperfecta	VZV	varicella zoster virus
PACNS	primary angiitis of the central nervous system	WBC	white blood cell
		WCC	white cell count
PAN	polyarteritis nodosa	WG	Wegener's granulomatosis (also known as granulomatosis with polyangiitis (GPA))
PAS	periodic acid–Schiff		
PCR	polymerase chain reaction		
PET	positron emission tomography		

Normal ranges

Haematology

haemoglobin	
males	g/L (130–180)
females	g/L (115–165)
MCV	fL (80–96)
white cell count	$\times 10^9$/L (4.0–11.0)
neutrophil count	$\times 10^9$/L (1.5–7.0)
lymphocyte count	$\times 10^9$/L (1.5–4.0)
monocyte count	$\times 10^9$/L (<0.8)
eosinophil count	$\times 10^9$/L (0.04–0.40)
platelet count	$\times 10^9$/L (150–400)
CD4 count	$\times 10^6$/L (430–1690)
erythrocyte sedimentation rate	
under 50 years:	
males	mm/ h (<15)
females	mm/ h (<20)
over 50 years:	
males	mm/ h (<20)
females	mm/ h (<30)

Haematinics

serum iron	µmol/L (12–30)
serum iron-binding capacity	µmol/L (45–75)
serum ferritin	µg/L (15–300)
serum transferrin	g/L (2.0–4.0)

Chemistry

Blood

serum sodium	mmol/L (137–144)
serum potassium	mmol/L (3.5–4.9)
serum creatinine	µmol/L (60–110)
estimated glomerular filtration rate	mL/min (>60)
serum corrected calcium	mmol/L (2.20–2.60)

serum total protein	g/L (61–76)
serum albumin	g/L (37–49)
serum globulin	g/L (24–27)
serum alanine aminotransferase	U/L (5–35)
serum alkaline phosphatase	U/L (45–105)
serum gamma glutamyl transferase	
males	U/L (<50)
females	U/L (4–35)
serum lactate dehydrogenase	U/L (10–250)
serum creatine kinase (CPK)	
males	U/L (24–195)
females	U/L (24–170)
fasting plasma glucose	mmol/L (3.0–6.0)
serum urate	
males	mmol/L (0.23–0.46)
females	mmol/L (0.19–0.36)
serum angiotensin-converting enzyme	U/L (25–82)

Urine

glomerular filtration rate	mL/min (70–140)
24-h urinary total protein	g (<0.2)

Lipids and lipoproteins

serum cholesterol	mmol/L (<5.2)
serum LDL cholesterol	mmol/L (<3.36)
serum HDL cholesterol	mmol/L (>1.55)
fasting serum triglycerides	mmol/L (0.45–1.69)

Thyroid hormones

plasma thyroid-binding globulin	mg/L (13–28)
plasma T4	nmol/L (58–174)
plasma parathyroid hormone	pmol/L (0.9–5.4)
serum cholecalciferol (vitamin D_3)	nmol/L (60–105)
serum 25-OH-cholecalciferol	nmol/L (45–90)
serum 1,25-$(OH)_2$-cholecalciferol	pmol/L (43–149)

Immunology

serum complement C3	mg/dL (65–190)
serum complement C4	mg/dL (15–50)

C-reactive protein (CRP)	mg/L (<8)
serum immunoglobulin G	g/L (6.0–13.0)
serum immunoglobulin A	g/L (0.8–3.0)
serum immunoglobulin M	g/L (0.4–2.5)

Autoantibodies

anticentromere antibodies	(negative at 1:40 dilution)
anticardiolipin antibodies:	
immunoglobulin G	U/mL (<23)
immunoglobulin M	U/mL (<11)
anti-cyclic citrullinated peptide antibodies (ACPA)	
anti-double-stranded DNA antibodies (ELISA)	U/mL (<73)
anti-neutrophil cytoplasmic antibodies:	
c-ANCA	
p-ANCA	
PR3-ANCA	U/mL (<10)
MPO-ANCA	U/mL (<10)
antinuclear antibodies	(negative at 1:20 dilution)
extractable nuclear antigen	
anti-Jo-1 antibodies	
anti-La antibodies	
antimitochondrial antibodies	(negative at 1:20 dilution)
anti-RNP antibodies	
anti-Scl-70 antibodies	
anti-Ro antibodies	
anti-Sm antibodies	
anti-smooth muscle antibodies	(negative at 1:20 dilution)
anti-thyroid colloid and microsomal antibodies	(negative at 1:10 dilution)
rheumatoid factor	kIU/L (<30)

Case 1

A 76-year-old widow presented to the Emergency Department with a mid-shaft right femoral fracture after a low-impact fall outside a supermarket. She had a past history of ischaemic heart disease, peripheral vascular disease, intermittent claudication, and mechanical right knee pain. She had been reviewed in rheumatology outpatients 3 months prior to admission for investigation of a painful swollen right elbow. She lived alone and had moved from County Durham where her husband had been a coal miner. Her usual medication included aspirin, bendroflumethiazide, and simvastatin.

On examination, in addition to the fractured femur she had a warm swollen R distal upper arm. She was haemodynamically stable, normotensive, and in sinus rhythm. Her distal pedal pulses were all impalpable.

Her initial blood results showed the following:

- Hb 10.5 g/dL (MCV 88 fL); WCC 6.8×10^9/L; platelets 468×10^9/L
- Creatinine 138 μmol/L; asparatate transaminase (AST) 48 IU/L; gamma glutamyl transferase (GGT) 52 IU/L; ALP 785 IU/L
- Corrected calcium 2.23 mmol/L; phosphate 1.2 mmol/L
- C-reactive protein (CRP) 8 mg/L.

Her femoral fracture was successfully pinned and plated, and she made a good post-operative recovery. Prior to discharge she was given an intravenous infusion. One week after discharge she was re-admitted profoundly unwell with nausea, vomiting, and tingling in her hands and feet.

Second admission bloods were as follows.

- Hb 11.5 g/dL (MCV 88 fL); WCC 7.9×10^9/L; platelets 488×10^9/L
- Creatinine 144 μmol/L; asparatate transaminase (AST) 55 IU/L; gamma glutamyl transferase (GGT) 30 IU/L; ALP189 IU/L
- CRP 10 mg/L
- Corrected calcium 1.87 mmol/L; phosphate 0.8 mmol/L
- Vitamin D level 7 nmol/L (threshold 20).

Radiographic findings are shown in Figs 1.1, 1.2, 1.3 and 1.4

Questions

1. What is the underlying bony diagnosis? What is the differential diagnosis? Describe the radiographic features in Figs 1.1–1.4.

2. Describe the clinical features, natural history, and potential complications of this condition.

3. What is the likely infusion she was given?

4. What complication of treatment did she develop and why?

5. Her daughter accompanies her to appointments and asks if she is likely to have this condition?

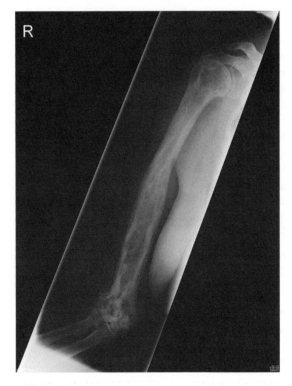

Fig. 1.1 Right humerus.

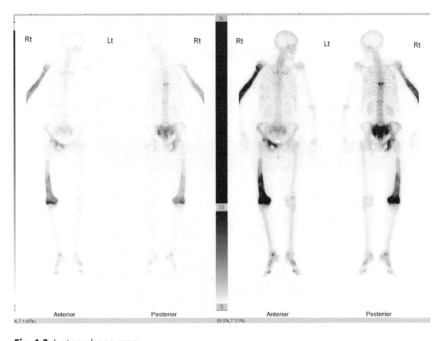

Fig. 1.2 Isotope bone scan.

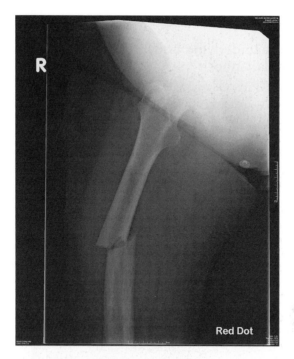

Fig. 1.3 Right femoral mid-shaft fracture.

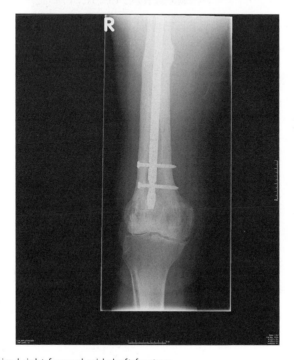

Fig. 1.4 Repaired right femoral mid-shaft fracture.

Answers

1. What is the underlying bony diagnosis? What is the differential diagnosis?

The diagnosis is Paget's disease of bone.

The differential diagnosis of a low-impact fracture in an elderly woman includes osteoporosis, osteomalacia, pathological fracture through a malignant focus, and Paget's disease. This patient's calcium was low normal on admission. Her phosphate was also low normal and her alkaline phosphate was very high. The rise in ALP could have been due to Paget's disease, osteomalacia, malignancy, or her recent fracture.

The plain radiographic features in the humerus (Fig. 1.1), and below the femoral fracture site (Fig. 1.3) in this case are typical of Paget's disease (Fig. 1.5). The bones are expanded with coarse trabeculation, cortical thickening, a mixture of lytic and sclerotic areas with intra-cortical resorption, loss of cortico-medullary junction, and early secondary osteoarthritis changes in the knee. Radiographic features are pathognomonic in established disease, but early or isolated lesions might be confused with malignancy and severe osteomalacia.

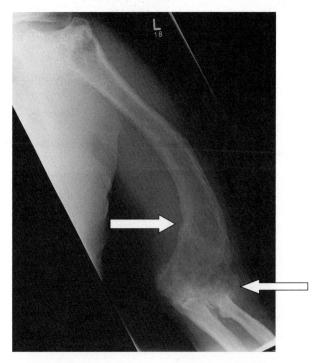

Fig. 1.5 Typical pagetic changes in a humerus with disorganized architecture, coarse trabeculation, cortical thickening, bowing and fractures in the cortex (arrow), and osteoarthritic changes in elbow (arrow) and shoulder.

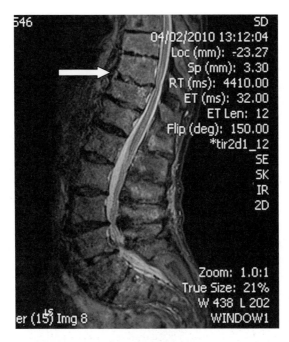

Fig. 1.6 MRI spine with spinal cord compression (arrow) and multi-level degeneration.

The technetium-99m isotope bone scan (Fig. 1.2) shows increased uptake in the right humerus right distal femur, right hemi-pelvis, and thoracic spine.

Isotope bone scans are the current standard method of establishing the pattern of skeletal site involvement. Typical abnormalities are easily recognized. However, if abnormalities are detected, further clinical and radiographic assessment is necessary. There is a move towards limited skeletal survey, imaging the clinically significant sites of skull, long bones, and spine as first-line investigation.

In this patient's technetium scan the characteristic V-shaped advancing front of Paget's disease is seen in the femur and humerus. This represents marked osteolysis without accompanying sclerosis. Other affected areas include the sacrum and the T9 vertebral body.

CT imaging may be useful to delineate difficult fractures and MRI should be used to characterize spinal Paget's disease which may cause nerve root compression and spinal canal stenosis (Fig. 1.6).

2. Describe the clinical features, natural history, and potential complications of this condition

Paget's disease of bone occurs in up to 10% of the population aged over 80 years and can affect any bone. The most common bones affected are pelvis (75%), lumbar spine (50%), femur (35%), sacrum (35%), skull (35%), tibia (30%) radius (15%). Patients often present with pain or deformity. The pain is of a deep bony, boring quality, and is present at rest. If the pagetic lesions involve subchondral bone they may result in secondary osteoarthritic changes and additional mechanical pain.

Pagetic bone is often increased in size, bowed, and mechanically weak. The bones are hypervascular, warm, and prone to fracture. Bony enlargement in the spine may cause mechanical compression of the nerve roots or spinal canal, leading to radicular pain or spinal claudication. Microfracture and vertebral collapse may lead to pain and kyphosis. The cause of pain may be difficult to determine and requires careful history and examination.

This patient's fracture is just above her pagetic bone and a typical site for pathological fracture. Prior to the fracture, her most troublesome symptom was her knee pain, attributed to associated osteoarthritis. As with many elderly patients, she has a number of comorbidities, including vascular claudication, which may have complicated the clinical picture.

Pagetic bone is hypervascular, and this has important consequences in relation to joint replacement surgery or surgery after fracture. The bleeding from hypervascular pagetic bone needs to be anticipated and is often difficult to control. Pretreatment with bisphosphonates may help prevent perioperative blood loss (see below). High-output cardiac failure, although often cited, is rarely seen in practice.

Deformity and associated symptoms are site-specific. Skull involvement can cause deafness from cranial nerve VIII compression, change in head shape, deep-seated headache, toothache (mandible involvement); blindness from optic nerve compression, and change in voice from nasal bone and airway narrowing. Long bones such as the tibia ('sabre tibia') and femur may be bowed, warm, and painful. Associated leg-length inequalities can lead to mechanical low back pain. Spinal involvement may lead to pain, spinal claudication; radicular symptoms from nerve root entrapment, or vertebral collapse and kyphosis.

Many patients are asymptomatic and Paget's disease is an incidental finding on X-ray or from a raised alkaline phosphatase (ALP) as part of a routine blood screen for liver function. The natural history is unknown. Patients may be asymptomatic for many years, and it is not yet known whether treatment of asymptomatic patients increases longevity or prevents future problems. However, treatment is generally given for lower-limb long-bone, spinal, skull, and painful pagetic lesions.

3. What is the likely infusion she was given?

This patient was treated with a potent intravenous bisphosphonate, either pamidronate or zoledronate.

The treatment of symptomatic Paget's disease of bone has been improved by the introduction of bisphosphonates which are potent inhibitors of bone turnover. The current regimes include 2 months oral risedronate 35 mg daily or 6 months oral alendronate 40 mg, quarterly intravenous pamidronate 30–90 mg over 2 h, or annual zolendronate 5 mg over 30 min. The aim of bisphosphonate therapy is to decrease pain, prevent further fracture, and normalize the alkaline phophatase. This is particularly effective prior to orthopaedic operations. Although there is a theoretical risk of impeding bone healing and remodelling by preventing osteoclast function, it is acceptable practice to use bisphosphonate therapy to try to prevent disease complications such as long-bone fracture.

ALP is the most commonly used marker of bisphosphonate activity. Bone resorption markers such as urinary cross-linked N-telopeptides of type 1 collagen (NTX) and serum carboxy-terminal collagen crosslinks (CTX) are raised, but are rarely helpful in clinical decision-making.

An ALP within the normal range may still be abnormally high for an individual patient, and comparison with premorbid ALP levels, if available, will help inform treatment decisions. In general, high ALP levels are associated with high disease activity.

Oral bisphosphonate normalizes ALP in 60% of patients at 18 months, IV pamidronate normalizes ALP in 50% at 6 months, and IV zoledronate normalizes ALP in 80% of patients at 6 months.

There is no benefit in terms of subsequent fracture rate or quality of life in treating Paget's disease to maintain normal ALP levels. Treatments are repeated according to patient symptoms. As yet there are no data about the safety and efficacy of long-term bisphosphonate use.

Patients who are intolerant of bisphosphonates may respond to calcitonin given by subcutaneous injection—100 units daily for 3–6 months. This treatment should reduce pain and ALP in up to 50% of patients at 6 months. Side effects, including flushing, nausea, and headache, are common and may limit therapy.

4. What complication of treatment did she develop and why?

This patient developed profound hypocalcaemia in the presence of previously undiagnosed hypovitaminosis D. Hypovitaminosis D is very common and under-diagnosed in the elderly, particularly from northern latitudes. Low vitamin D levels can lead to myalgia, bone pain, weakness, and even falls. Borderline vitamin D levels in this woman prior to bisphosphonate infusion exaggerated the hypocalcaemic effect and led to dangerously low serum calcium levels.

All bisphosphonates can cause hypocalcaemia. The effect is greater with the more powerful longer-acting preparations and in patients with low vitamin D levels. Ideally, all patients should have their serum calcium and vitamin D levels checked before administration of parenteral bisphosphonate. As vitamin D levels are not always readily available, it is recommended that all patients receiving bisphosphonate treatment should receive calcium and vitamin D supplementation unless there are specific contraindications.

Oral bisphosphonate preparations need to be taken on an empty stomach with a large glass of water, and the patient should remain upright for at least 30 minutes before eating. Gastritis and indigestion are common. Many centres are moving towards using the more powerful longer-acting intra-venous preparations because of poor compliance and gastrointestinal side effects with the oral preparations. This general move is mirrored in the treatment of osteoporosis, where there is widespread use of bisphosphonates. Therefore this case serves to illustrate a potential problem that could occur with increasing use of powerful long-acting bisphosphonates.

5. Her daughter accompanies her to appointments and asks if she is likely to have this condition?

Paget's disease of bone commonly occurs in families with an autosomal dominant but incompletely penetrant pattern of inheritance. As a first-degree relative, this woman's daughter has a seven times increased risk of developing the condition.

There is ethnic and geographic clustering around cooler latitudes, particularly Europe, North America, and Australasia. The highest prevalence is in populations from northern Britain and where they have subsequently migrated into the former British colonies.

Recent genetic studies from familial Paget's disease of bone have linked a number of genetic loci and mutations have been identified in four genes, the most important of which is sequestosome 1 (SQSTM1). This is a scaffold protein in the nuclear factor kappa B (NFkappaB) signalling pathway. Patients with SQSTM1 mutations have severe Paget's disease with a high degree of penetrance with increasing age. Environmental factors, such as deficiency in dietary calcium, and repeated mechanical loading have recently been linked to Paget's disease of bone. Other possible environmental triggers include paramyxoviral infection, measles, canine distemper, and respiratory syncytial virus. Given the ubiquitous nature of many of these viruses, interplay of genetic and environmental factors must occur to explain the geographical distribution as well as the focal and heterogenous nature of the condition.

Further reading

Cooper MS, Gittoes NJ (2008). Diagnosis and management of hypocalcaemia. *BMJ*; **336**: 1298–1302.

Langston AL, Campbell MK, Fraser WD, *et al.* (2010). Randomized trial of intensive bisphosphonate treatment versus symptomatic management in Paget's disease of bone. *J Bone Miner Res*; **25**: 20–31.

Mouyis M Ostor AJ, Crisp AJ, *et al.* (2008). Hypovitaminosis D among rheumatology outpatients in clinical practice. *Rheumatology*; **47**: 1348–51.

Paget, J. (1877). On a form of chronic inflammation of bones (osteitis deformans). *Trans Med-Chir Soc*; **60**: 235–56.

Peter R, Mishra V, Fraser WD (2007). Severe hypocalcaemia after being given intravenous bisphosphonate. *BMJ*; **328**: 335–6.

Scarsbrook A, Brown M, Wilson D (2004).UK guidelines on management of Paget's disease of bone. *Rheumatology*; **43**: 399–400.

Siris ES, Lyles KW, Singer FR, Meunier PJ (2006). Medical management of Paget's disease of the bone: indications for treatment and review of current therapies. *J Bone Miner Res*; **21** (Suppl 2): 94–8.

Soni A, Williamson L (2008). Paget's disease—limited skeletal survey may be better than isotope bone scan; an inconvenient truth? *Clin Radiol*; **63**: 108–10.

Case 2

A 60-year-old woman was referred to the lymphoma clinic in view of a 2 month history of night sweats, fatigue, and general malaise. There was no past medical or travel history of note, but significant weight loss had been noted by her husband. She denied any gastrointestinal symptoms but had been experiencing recurrent generalized headaches over the last 6 weeks. She was a lifelong non-smoker and drank alcohol only occasionally.

On examination she had a temperature of 38.2°C, but other vital signs were normal. She appeared thin with no lymphadenopathy. Full systemic examination, including urinalysis, was otherwise normal.

Investigations revealed elevated inflammatory markers (erythrocyte sedimentation rate (ESR) 85 mm/h, CRP 44 mg/L) but no evidence of haematological abnormality, infection, or malignancy. The results of diagnostic and staging investigations are shown in Figs 2.1 and 2.2, respectively.

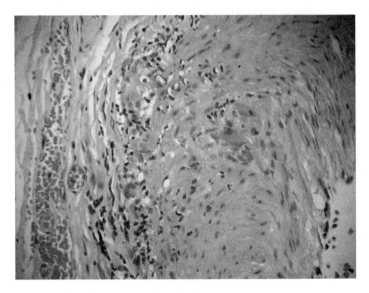

Fig. 2.1 (See also Plate 1) Diagnostic investigation.

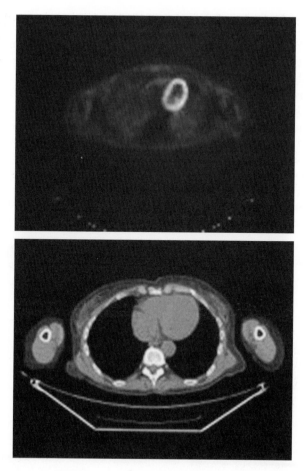

Fig. 2.2 Staging investigation.

Questions

1. What is the diagnosis? What is the diagnostic investigation that was performed and what abnormalities are shown in Fig. 2.1?

2. Which investigation results are shown in Fig. 2.2? When should this investigation be considered?

3. What is the most worrying complication of this condition?

4. What features should be sought on examination?

5. What immediate action should be taken when this condition is suspected?

6. Which other imaging modality may be helpful in the investigation of this condition?

Answers

1. What is the diagnosis? What is the diagnostic investigation that was performed and what abnormalities are shown in Fig. 2.1?

The diagnosis is giant cell arteritis (GCA), also known as temporal arteritis or Horton's headache. It is a primary large vessel vasculitis with a mean age at onset of 70 years. It is rare before the age of 50 years and is more common in Caucasian than African Caribbean people. It has a significant female preponderance. Headache is the most common complaint; it occurs in 90% of patients and is the presenting feature in 48% of cases. Headaches can be quite variable in quality and nature, and can mimic tension headache, migraine, and cluster headaches. Other common features include scalp tenderness and jaw or tongue claudication. Systemic features including fever, weight loss, and malaise occur in 50% of patients. Rarely, it can present with systemic features alone or limb claudication.

The diagnostic investigation is a temporal artery biopsy (Figs 2.1 and 2.3). This investigation should be considered in all cases of suspected temporal arteritis. Ideally, a temporal artery biopsy should be obtained within a week of commencing steroids in order to maximize its diagnostic and prognostic value. However, there is evidence to suggest that temporal artery biopsy may remain positive up to 28 days after commencing steroid therapy. Contralateral biopsy does not provide any additional information and is not routinely recommended. In order to maximize the diagnostic potential, a biopsy at least 1 cm long is suggested. This example (Fig. 2.3) demonstrates the classical histological features of GCA which include:

- disruption of the internal elastic membrane (1)
- multinucleate giant cells (2)
- occlusion of the lumen (3)
- intimal hyperplasia (4).

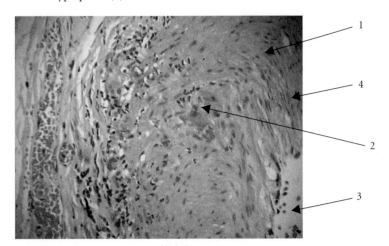

Fig. 2.3 (See also Plate 2) Temporal artery biopsy.

The severity of intimal hyperplasia on temporal artery biopsy is associated with increased risk of neuro-ophthalmic complications.

2. Which investigation results are shown in Fig. 2.2? When should this investigation be considered?

Figure 2.2 shows the results of a whole-body FDG PET scan. The use of FDG, a glucose analogue, enables the visualization of inflamed vessels, which are glucose-consuming, provided that they are greater than 4 mm in diameter. This size limitation and proximity to the high glucose consumption of the brain explains why the temporal arteries themselves are not visible using this imaging modality. Large-vessel vasculitis can be demonstrated and is particularly specific to large-vessel vasculitis when seen in the larger thoracic vessels, as is seen here with marked aortitis.

This type of imaging should be considered in patients demonstrating systemic features, limb claudication, or persistent symptoms despite adequate steroid therapy. MRI can also be used to assess for large-vessel involvement and does not expose the patient to radiation.

3. What is the most worrying complication of this condition?

Visual loss is the most serious complication of GCA, and occurs in 15% of patients. If one eye is affected, there is high risk (20–50%) of bilateral loss of vision if there is any delay or cessation of treatment. Blindness is most commonly the result of optic ischaemic neuropathy and is associated with a positive temporal artery biopsy. Retinal and ophthalmic artery thromboses are rare causes of blindness in GCA.

4. What features should be sought on examination?

Examination findings include the following:

♦ **Cranial**: tender, thickened, or beaded superficial temporal artery with reduced or absent pulsation, scalp tenderness, and upper cranial nerve palsies.

♦ **Visual**: transient or permanent reduction in acuity, relative afferent pupillary defect, and pale swollen optic disc.

♦ **Systemic**: asymmetrical pulses and blood pressure, presence of bruits.

The presence of temporal artery prominence, beading, and tenderness all increase the likelihood of obtaining a positive temporal artery biopsy.

5. What immediate action should be taken when this condition is suspected?

All patients with suspected GCA should be commenced on high-dose steroids immediately. The dose and administration of steroids depends on the clinical scenario.

♦ Uncomplicated GCA with no claudication or visual symptoms: 40–60 mg daily.

♦ Evolving visual loss or amaurosis fugax: intravenous methylprednisolone 500 mg for 3 days before commencing oral steroids.

♦ Established visual loss: 60 mg prednisolone daily, to protect the contralateral eye.

All patients should receive bone protection with calcium and vitamin D supplements and a bisphosphonate (see p. 7). Gastric protection with a proton pump inhibitor should also be considered. Once the diagnosis has been confirmed, aspirin is recommended if no contraindication exists, and statin therapy can also be considered. Steroid-sparing agents, such as methotrexate or azathioprine, may be indicated if there is evidence of recurrent relapse or difficulty weaning steroids.

Essential investigations include full blood count, liver function tests, urea and electrolytes, ESR, CRP, and urgent temporal artery biopsy. These investigations should not delay initiation of appropriate treatment.

6. Which other imaging modality may be helpful in the investigation of this condition?

The diagnostic use of ultrasound in GCA is currently under investigation. It is widely available, relatively inexpensive, repeatable, non-invasive, and lacks radiation exposure. It can provide information regarding the vessel wall, lumen, pulsatility, and blood flow characteristics. The main potential drawback of ultrasound is operator dependency, although recent studies of temporal artery ultrasound have shown inter-observer agreement of more than 90%.

The features shown on ultrasound include the following:

◆ **Oedema**: a dark hypoechoic thickening or halo around the vessel wall.

◆ **Stenosis**: manifests as disrupted turbulent blood flow on colour Doppler.

◆ **Occlusion**: colour signals are absent.

A recent meta-analysis showed that temporal artery ultrasonography has a pooled sensitivity of 80% and specificity of 96% compared with the clinical diagnosis. Further studies are under way to explore this further and determine the pragmatic utility of ultrasound in the diagnosis of GCA.

Further reading

Blockmans D, Bley T, Schmidt W (2009). Imaging for large-vessel vasculitis. *Curr Opin Rheumatol*; **21**: 19–28.

Mukhtyar C, Guillevin L, Cid MC, *et al.* (2009). EULAR recommendations for the management of large vessel vasculitis. *Ann Rheum Dis*; **68**: 318–23.

Case 3

A 19-year-old Brazilian woman, who was previously well, presented with a 10-day history of sudden-onset polyarthritis and a diffuse necrotizing rash. Since moving to England 4 years previously, she had noticed nasal congestion and clear discharge during the winter months. Examination revealed fever (37.9°C), tachycardia (110 beats/min), tender axillary and inguinal lymphadenopathy, and a symmetrical synovitis of elbows, wrists, ankles, and MCP joints. She had widespread tender erythematous nodules over her face, arms, and legs with truncal sparing (Fig. 3.1).

Investigations showed the following:

◆ CRP 191 mg/L

◆ Routine biochemistry, FBC, RF, ANA, ANCA, complement levels, CPK, throat swab, ASOT, Epstein–Barr virus (EBV), and cytomegalovirus (CMV) serology, urine microscopy, and three sets of blood cultures were all normal

◆ ECG showed sinus tachycardia

◆ CXR normal

◆ Skin biopsy initially showed granulomatous and perivascular inflammation (Fig. 3. 2).

By day 5 of admission, the patient became increasingly unwell with persistent pyrexia, and worsening periorbital inflammation. She also developed numbness in a stocking distribution with preserved reflexes and power. In response to the clinical deterioration empirical treatment with intravenous methylprednisolone was administered.

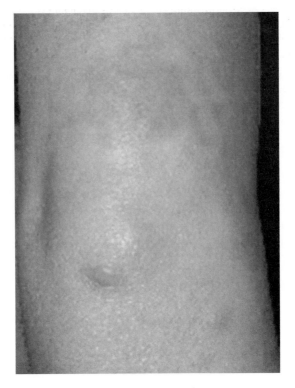

Fig. 3.1 (See also Plate 3) Erythematous nodules on elbow.

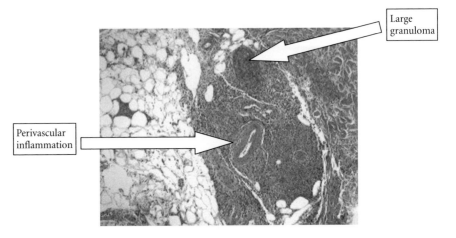

Fig. 3.2 (See also Plate 4) Skin biopsy with haematoxylin and eosin staining.

Questions

1. What is the differential diagnosis based on the clinical features?
2. The initial skin biopsy (Fig. 3.2) shows granulomatous inflammation. How does this alter the differential diagnosis?

Answers

1. What is the differential diagnosis based on the clinical features?

The presence of a rash and small-joint polyarthritis raises a broad differential. Primary rheumatological conditions would include systemic lupus erythematosis, which would be supported by the malar distribution of the rash, dermatomyositis, which can cause severe periorbital oedema, and vasculitis, with the nasal discharge. Wegener's granulomatosis (WG) should be considered (see p. 131). In addition, the history should be explored for features of a possible reactive arthritis (see p. 249) or a drug reaction.

The presence of fever and tender nodules on the face raise the possibility of acute febrile neutrophilic dermatosis or Sweet's syndrome. This is characterized by tender red-to-purple papules, and nodules that coalesce to form plaques usually on the upper extremities, face, and neck. It is due to a hypersensitivity reaction in response to systemic factors such as haematological disease, infection, inflammation, vaccination, or drug exposure. However, the condition is mediated by neutrophils and therefore is not supported in the current case by the normal peripheral white cell count.

2. The initial skin biopsy (Fig. 3.2) shows granulomatous inflammation. How does this alter the differential diagnosis?

The skin biopsy with haematoxylin and eosin staining shows evidence of perivascular necrotizing granulomatous inflammation. Larger magnification also revealed perineural inflammation.

The presence of granulomatous inflammation on the skin biopsy is still in keeping with vasculitis, in particular WG. Lymphomatoid granulomatosis, an angio-destructive lymphoproliferative systemic disease associated with EBV which is known to mimic WG, should also be considered but is less likely in the context of the negative serology. Granulomatous disease in the context of musculoskeletal symptoms should always raise the possibility of sarcoidosis (see p. 20) and its counterpart tuberculosis. A normal chest X-ray (CXR) does not exclude either of these diagnoses. Alongside tuberculosis, another granulomatous infectious aetiology is leprosy.

The absence of a neutrophilic inflammatory response, in addition to the normal peripheral white cell count, excludes the diagnosis of Sweet's syndrome.

Further staining revealed the presence of acid-fast bacilli on Wade–Fite staining, diagnostic of leprosy (Fig. 3.3).

3. What are the musculoskeletal manifestations of leprosy?

Musculoskeletal complications are common and include arthralgia, arthritis, and Charcot joints. A symmetrical small-joint polyarthritis, mimicking rheumatoid arthritis, is common, and the combination of arthritis, neurological involvement, and skin lesions can easily be misdiagnosed as primary vasculitis. The subsequent

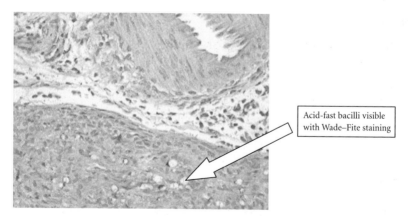

Acid-fast bacilli visible
with Wade–Fite staining

Fig. 3.3 (See also Plate 5) Skin biopsy with Wade–Fite staining.

delay in diagnosis can be a number of years, even in countries with endemic leprosy such as India. Untreated leprosy results in severely reduced quality of life, mainly due to diffuse irreversible nerve damage. Moreover, the use of systemic immuno-suppressive agents for a presumed non-infective condition can impact on the disease activity and progression to the more severe lepromatous form of leprosy.

Further reading

Cossermelli-Messina W, Festa, Neto C, Cossermelli W (1998). Articular inflammatory manifestations in patients with different forms of leprosy. *J Rheumatol*; **25**: 111–19.

Haroon N, Agarwal V, Aggarwal A, Kumari N, Krishnani N, Misra R (2007). Arthritis as presenting manifestation of pure neuritic leprosy—a rheumatologist's dilemma. *Rheumatology*; **46**: 653–6.

Case 4

A 32-year-old Caucasian primary school teacher was seen in the rheumatology clinic. Eight weeks previously she had developed generalized malaise and a sore throat. These symptoms resolved within a week, but 3 weeks later she developed a rash over the dorsum of her feet and shins. The rash comprised multiple red tender lumps. She also developed pain and swelling of both ankles, alongside mild aching of the limb girdle. The joint symptoms improved slightly with naproxen, prescribed by her general practitioner. She had no significant travel history.

On examination she appeared systemically well, with mild swelling and tenderness of both ankles. The rash had resolved apart from a single yellowish tender lesion on her right shin. The rest of her examination was normal.

Investigations showed the following:

- FBC, U&Es, LFTs, calcium, CPK, TSH all normal
- CRP 36 mg/L, ESR 24 mm/h
- ASOT 20 U/ml.

The CXR is shown in Fig. 4.1.

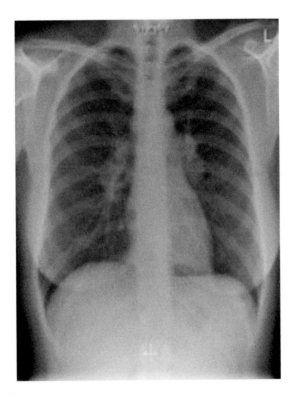

Fig. 4.1 Chest X-ray.

Questions

1. What is the rash likely to be and what is the differential diagnosis, based on the history and examination findings alone?

2. What is the most likely diagnosis, taking the CXR findings into account?

3. What is a likely explanation for this patient's muscle aches and what are the systemic manifestations of this condition?

4. How would you manage this patient and what is her prognosis?

Answers

1. What is the rash likely to be and what is the differential diagnosis, based on the history and examination findings alone?

The rash is most likely to be due to erythema nodosum. It characteristically develops as an acute nodular erythematous eruption. It is most commonly found on the extensor aspect of the legs and is particularly painful during the first week. As it heals, it changes from red to blue and ultimately resembles a bruise. Individual lesions tend to last for about 2 weeks, but individual crops usually develop in a staggered fashion.

The presence of a sore throat prior to the onset of the joint symptoms raises the possibility of rheumatic fever or a post-streptococcal reactive arthritis (see p. 249). The arthritis of rheumatic fever does usually affect large joints, including the knees and ankles, and usually settles within 1–2 weeks. However, the absence of the typical migratory polyarthritis, whereby several joints are affected in quick succession, each for a brief period of time, makes it unlikely. It would also usually be accompanied by an acute febrile illness. Although it is possible that the nodular rash represents the subcutaneous nodules found in rheumatic fever, these tend to be painless and resolve within a few days. The presentation is not typical for post-streptococcal reactive arthritis either, as it usually develops 2 weeks after the initial throat infection and is often associated with a non-migratory large-joint oligoarthritis which persists for longer than 2 weeks.

Reactive arthritis does commonly affect the ankles and many of the causative organisms, including *Mycoplasma*, *Campylobacter*, and *Salmonella*, are also associated with erythema nodosum. However, there is nothing in this patient's history to suggest a preceding infective illness with these organisms.

Viral arthritis (see p. 246), for example following human parvovirus B19 infection, is another possibility: particularly given that the patient is a primary school teacher. However, the viral arthritides tend to develop during the viral prodrome itself and are usually associated with a symmetrical small-joint polyarthritis, with a predilection for the upper limbs.

Other causes of arthritis or arthralgia in the context of erythema nodosum include enteropathic arthritis (see p. 31), Behçet's disease (BD), lymphoma, tuberculosis, and acute sarcoidosis. Although enteropathic arthritis does usually result in a large-joint oligoarthritis affecting the knees and ankles, this woman does not have any symptoms suggestive of underlying inflammatory bowel disease (IBD). BD (see p. 223) would be uncommon in a Caucasian female, and it is usually associated with orogenital ulceration. Arthritis as the presenting feature of lymphoma in adults is rare, and has been reported more in children. Tuberculosis can spread to affect joints by haematogenous or lymphatic routes, or via contiguous spread from an infected area. This tends to affect the spine and large weight-bearing joints. Alternatively, pulmonary or other organ tuberculosis can cause a reactive polyarthritis known as Poncet's disease. This can affect any joint areas, but knees, ankles, and elbows are the most common. This patient does not have any known risk factors or symptoms suggestive of tuberculosis. Patients with acute sarcoidosis commonly have joint complaints (50%), with symmetrical ankle involvement being a strong diagnostic indicator.

2. What is the most likely diagnosis, taking the CXR findings into account?

The CXR shows right paratracheal lymphadenopathy with symmetrical bilateral hilar lymphadenopathy. These radiographic findings comprise Garland's triad, which is a commonly seen in sarcoidosis with pulmonary involvement. Chest radiograph findings are staged as follows.

- Stage 0: Normal
- Stage 1: Bilateral hilar lymphadenopathy
- Stage 2: Bilateral hilar lymphadenopathy with parenchymal involvement
- Stage 3: Parenchymal involvement with shrinking adenopathy
- Stage 4: Parenchymal involvement evolves to show volume loss.

As there is no parenchymal involvement, this would be consistent with stage 1 disease. Lymphoma is an important differential diagnosis in the context of bilateral hilar lymphadenopathy, and can only be definitively excluded on biopsy.

Therefore the most likely diagnosis is acute sarcoidosis with stage 1 pulmonary involvement.

3. What is a likely explanation for this patient's muscle aches and what are the systemic manifestations of this condition?

Muscle involvement in sarcoidosis is relatively common, occurring in 50–80% of cases. It is usually asymptomatic and so is often undetected. Granulomatous muscle involvement can lead to weakness, proximal pain, and tenderness. This may be focal or diffuse, in which case it is symmetrical and causes progressive weakness and atrophy. Electromyography (EMG) studies show similar findings to polymyositis.

Sarcoidosis is a multisystemic condition of unknown aetiology, characterized by the presence of non-caseating granuloma in affected tissues. The various manifestations are summarized below:

- Lungs (90%):
  - lymphadenopathy
  - parenchymal involvement
  - pleural involvement may manifest as pneumothorax or pleural effusion (rare).
- Skin (25%):
  - erythema nodosum
  - subcutaneous nodules
  - papules

- plaques
- lupus pernio.
◆ Joints (50%):
  - transient flitting arthralgia can precede fever
  - symmetrical periarthritis
  - knees, ankles.
◆ Bone (30%):
  - cysts, hands, and feet
  - lytic lesions (rare) in the vertebral bodies, and occasionally in skull, long bones.
◆ Eyes (25%):
  - keratoconjunctivitis
  - uveitis
  - retinal vasculitis.
◆ Neurological (5%):
  - unilateral facial nerve palsy
  - hypothalamic–pituitary axis
  - basal granulomatous infiltration
  - peripheral neuropathy.
◆ Abdominal (50%):
  - hepatosplenomegaly
  - nephrolithiasis due to hypercalcaemia.
◆ Cardiac (5%):
  - cor pulmonale due to lung disease
  - arrhythmia
  - left ventricular failure
  - pericarditis.

4. How would you manage this patient and what is her prognosis?

The joint symptoms usually improve with a combination of rest and non-steroidal anti-inflammatory drug (NSAID) treatment. In severe cases, steroids or colchicine may be used, but there is little evidence base for this.

Pulmonary involvement is treated according to disease and symptom severity. Steroid therapy is first line in symptomatic disease. Although stage 4 disease represents pulmonary fibrosis, patients usually still derive symptomatic benefit which may be due to suppression of ongoing inflammation. In resistant cases, immunosuppressive agents have been used with variable benefit, but lung transplantation should be considered in those with progressive treatment-resistant disease.

The erythema nodosum usually self-resolves within a few weeks, but topical steroid therapy can be used as required.

Further reading

Visser H, Vos K, Zanelli E, *et al.* (2002). Sarcoid arthritis: clinical characteristics, diagnostic aspects, and risk factors. *Ann Rheum Dis*; **61**: 499–504.

Case 5

A 76-year-old retired general practitioner presented to the rheumatology department with polyarthritis which had developed insidiously over the previous 18 months. He was a lifelong asthmatic with a 10-year history of hypertension, a heavy smoker, and a heavy social drinker. He took diclofenac, enalapril, and prednisolone 5 mg daily, and used salbutamol and beclometasone inhalers. He admitted to self-medicating with oral steroids for most of his life to control his chest symptoms.

On examination, he was in atrial fibrillation and had a barrel-shaped chest. He had bilateral swelling of his MCP joints, a left knee effusion, a right olecranon bursa, Dupuytren's contractures, and signs consistent with right carpal tunnel syndrome.

Investigations showed the following:

- Hb 16 g/L; WCC 7×10^9/L; platelets 232×10^9/L

- Liver function normal; creatinine 135 µmol/L; glomerular filtration rate (GFR) 55; fasting glucose 5.5 mmol/L; urate 642 mmol/L

- CRP 10; RF latex screen positive; ELISA equivocal; anticitrullinated C-peptide (ACCP) negative.

Questions

1. What is the likely diagnosis and why?
2. Aspirate from the knee helped confirm the diagnosis. What are the likely findings?
3. What is the significance of the rheumatoid factor and uric acid levels?
4. What are the clinical manifestations of hyperuricaemia?
5. What management strategies will you suggest?

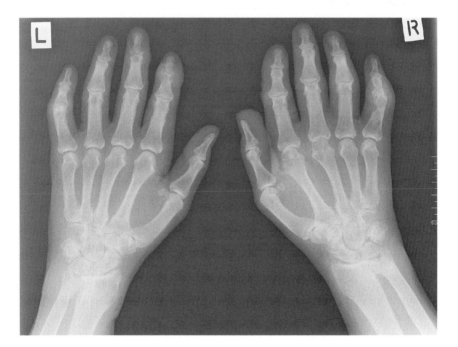

Fig. 5.1 X-ray of patient's hands.

Answers

1. What is the likely diagnosis and why?

The most likely diagnosis is chronic gout.

The differential diagnosis is between an acute inflammatory arthritis such as rheumatoid arthritis and chronic gout. The radiograph (Fig. 5.1) shows asymmetrical swelling with 'punched-out' erosions away from the joint surface with no osteopenia. The long-term steroid use is likely to have masked early episodic attacks of gout. Gout often affects osteoarthritic joints. Tophi over Heberden's or Bouchard's nodes can ulcerate and discharge, mimicking septic arthritis.

This patient could have developed an acute inflammatory arthritis in addition to long-standing chronic gout which had been masked by long-term steroid use. This is an important differential diagnosis to make as the management of the two conditions is very different.

2. Aspirate from the knee helped confirm the diagnosis. What are the likely findings?

Knee aspirate revealed negatively birefringent monosodium urate crystals. A diagnosis of gout is confirmed by the presence of uric acid crystals in a joint bursa or tophus. Aspirate from his olecranon bursa was thick, chalky, and rich in urate crystals.

Ideally, affected joints should be aspirated. However, if there are no actively inflamed joints, aspirate and washout from unaffected joints can aid diagnosis. The most common joint used in this situation is the knee. Diagnosis is confirmed if uric acid crystals are present in macrophages.

3. What is the significance of the rheumatoid factor and uric acid levels?

The rheumatoid factor is positive in approximately 10% of patients over the age of 60, and the percentage increases with age. The ACCP antibody is more specific for RA, and can help to differentiate between the two conditions. However, negative ACCP antibodies do not help to differentiate between gout and rheumatoid arthritis.

Hyperuricaemia does not equate to a diagnosis of gout. Furthermore, serum urate levels fall, and may be misleadingly low during attacks of gout. However, hyperuricaemia is the most important risk factor for developing acute gout, with a 5-year cumulative risk of one-third for patients with serum urate >0.6 mmol/L.

4. What are the clinical manifestations of hyperuricaemia?

The clinical manifestations of hyperuricaemia are:

- asymptomatic hyperuricaemia
- acute gout
- recurrent gout
- chronic tophaceous gout

- ◆ renal stone
- ◆ rarely urate nephropathy.

5. What management strategies will you suggest?

Gout is associated with hypertension, metabolic syndrome, insulin resistance, diabetes, and chronic renal failure.

Once a diagnosis of gout is established, the aims of management are to control symptoms, prevent future attacks, and prevent structural damage of joints and kidneys. This patient presents a number of management problems because of his long-term steroid use and comorbidities, including hypertension and borderline renal function.

NSAIDs should be stopped as they can exacerbate hypertension and decrease renal perfusion. In addition, the combination with oral corticosteroids puts this patient at high risk of a gastrointestinal bleed. Cyclo-oxgenase-2 (COX-2) selective NSAIDs such as etoricoxib and celecoxib have better gastrointestinal profiles, but should not be used in patients with pre-existing cardiovascular disease.

Oral colchicine at a dose of 500 μg twice to four times daily is an alternative treatment for inflammatory joint symptoms. Higher doses can cause diarrhoea. Simple analgesics should be used for pain relief. Intra-articular or intramuscular steroids can help settle the acute inflammatory symptoms.

For long-term control of joint symptoms, the serum urate needs to be lowered and maintained below the saturation point for monosodium urate (<0.38 mmol/L). Target levels for serum urate are <0.30 mmol/L (BSR) and < 0.36 mmol/L (European League Against Rheumatism (EULAR)).

Patients with gout are either under-excretors or over-producers of uric acid. This patient, as with 90% of patients, is likely to be an under-excretor of uric acid. Long-term treatment using uricostatic or uricosuric therapies is needed if patients are unable lower their serum urate sufficiently to prevent attacks of gout with lifestyle modification. This is especially so in renal failure patients with symptomatic gout. The long-term treatment of choice is prevention of urate production using allopurinol is a xanthine oxidase inhibitor which inhibits production of urate from hypoxanthine and xanthine. Allopurinol should be started once the acute symptoms have been settled for 2–6 weeks using colchicines (or NSAIDs if the patient is not in renal failure), otherwise there is a significant risk of acute gouty flare. The starting dose depends on the GFR (>80 mL/min, 300 mg daily; 15 mL/min, 50 mg on alternate days) This patient (GFR 60) should start at 100 mg daily and increase by 50 mg doses at fortnightly intervals until his serum urate is <0.030 mmol/L. Transient rashes (2%) are uncommon but usually settle with dose reduction. Rarely, a life-threatening allergic reaction with high fever, exfoliative dermatitis, acute hepatitis, interstitial nephritis, and vasculitis can occur. Desensitization regimes are possible, but are rarely used in practice.

Patients who are intolerant or allergic to allopurinol can use a uricosuric agent to enhance urate renal clearance. These drugs inhibit the urate anion exchange in the proximal nephron (URAT-1). Sulfinpyrazone (200–800 mg/day in divided doses) is the only drug readily available in the UK, but requires normal renal function. It is effective in diuretic-induced gout. Probenecid (0.5–2.0 g/day) can be used in mild renal failure (creatinine <200 mol/L) and is available on a named patient only basis in UK. Benzbromarone (50–200 mg/day) is effective in mild renal failure (eGFR 30–60) but is unlicensed in the UK (available on named patient basis). All three drugs have a significantly worse side-effect profile than allopurinol and are used as second-line agents in the UK. Benzbromarone can be used in combination with allopurinol.

Febuxostat (40–80 mg/day) is a recently developed non-purine selective xanthine oxidase inhibitor which is available to patients who are allergic to allopurinol and have failed uricosuric therapy.

Enzyme therapy with urate oxidase is now licensed for intravenous infusion treatment for allopurinol-intolerant patients. As a new therapy, the use will be limited by antibody formation and cost.

Lifestyle advice is important. Patients with early or mild gout can prevent future attacks by altering their lifestyle.

- Fluid intake depends on cardiovascular and renal function. In general, patients are advised to drink plenty of water to prevent renal stones. Over-producers of uric acid and those taking uricosuric agents are particularly prone to renal stones.

- Sweetened soft drinks and drinks high in fructose are associated with increased risk of gout in men.

- Dietary advice is the same as the general advice given for the associated metabolic syndrome. In addition, patients should avoid foods rich in purines such as red meat, game, offal, and shellfish.

- Alcohol enhances urate production, decreases renal urate clearance, decreases solubility of urate crystals, and can be relatively dehydrating. Beer, even non-alcoholic beer, is purine rich. Avoid beer and binge drinking. Limit alcohol intake per week to <21 units (men) and <14 units (women).

It is important to monitor renal function and general metabolic state. The patient's metabolic syndrome may be a much more serious cause of mortality and morbidity than their gout. The lipid-lowering drugs atorvostatin and fenofibrate, and the antihypertensives losartan and amlodipine, have mild uricosuric effects. This may be helpful when treating the comorbid conditions associated with gout.

Further reading

Jordan KM, Cameron JS, Snaith M, *et al.* (2007). British Society for Rheumatology and British Health Professionals in Rheumatology guideline for the management of chronic gout. *Rheumatology*; **46**: 1372–4.

Rider T, Jordan K (2010). The modern management of gout. *Rheumatology*; **49**: 5–14.

Zhang W, Doherty M, Bardin T, *et al.* (2006). EULAR evidence based recommendations for gout. *Ann Rheum Dis*; **65**: 1301–11.

Case 6

A 17-year-old Caucasian male was seen urgently in outpatients with a 3-week history of intermittent pain and swelling of his right knee. He had a past history of heel pain when he was 12 years old which had settled spontaneously. He was otherwise healthy, with no recent trauma and no significant past medical history. A paternal uncle had psoriasis.

On examination his height and weight were on the 60th centile and he was apyrexial with normal pulse and blood pressure. Examination of skin and musculoskeletal system was normal apart from a tense effusion of his right knee: 150 mL of straw-coloured fluid was aspirated from his knee and 80 mg of Depo-Medrone® was injected.

Investigations showed the following:

- Hb 12.4 g/dL; MCV 74 fL; WCC 12.4 × 10^9/L; neutrophils 6.9 × 10^9/L; platelets 488 × 10^9/L; CRP 89.2 mg/L
- Renal and liver functions were normal
- Synovial fluid: no organisms; no crystals; 2+ WCC; 0 RBC; no growth.

Questions—Part 1

1. What is the differential diagnosis?
2. What further information is needed to make the diagnosis?

Answers

1. What is the differential diagnosis?

In a young person, the most important differential diagnoses to consider are septic arthritis (see p. 208), trauma, and reactive arthritis. A travel history and sexual history are essential. With teenagers, it may be important to interview the patient without their parents to obtain an accurate history. The differential diagnosis is wide and includes enthesitis-related juvenile idiopathic arthritis (JIA), early seronegative inflammatory arthritis (psoriatic or enteropathic), undifferentiated spondylarthritis with peripheral joint involvement, atypical presentation of rheumatoid arthritis, and rarer conditions such as BD and acute sarcoidosis. In older patients a crystal arthritis should be considered.

Enthesitis-related JIA would fit with the previous history of heel pain and knee swelling, more common in human leucocyte antigen (HLA) B27-positive patients (his first rheumatological presentation was at age 12). The heel pain may represent an enthesopathy; these are frequently associated with spondyloarthritis but, as their symptoms are short-lived, they are often forgotten by patients and therefore need direct enquiry and examination.

The MCV of 74 fL is significant. Blood loss due to NSAID use, iron-deficiency anaemia due to malabsorption, inadequate diet, and blood loss should be considered. This patient had normal growth and was on the 60th centile for height and weight, which would not support a diagnosis of long-standing malabsorption. However, undiagnosed coeliac disease is known to be present in 0.5% of the population, and should be screened for. There is an association with muscle pain, probably related to low-grade vitamin D insufficiency. There is no association with inflammatory arthritis.

His low MCV might suggest a diagnosis of asymptomatic enteropathic arthritis.

A careful GI history, particularly noting mouth ulcers, weight loss, and systemic malaise should be obtained.

A history of psoriasis in a second-degree relative is of borderline significance, given the background population frequency of psoriasis; however, it does lend weight to a diagnosis of psoriatic arthritis. In younger children, a history of psoriasis in a first-degree relative (psoriatic diathesis) may be enough for a diagnosis of psoriatic arthritis, as the arthritis may precede the skin disease by many years, particularly in children.

2. What further information is needed to make the diagnosis?

A personal or family history of iritis, psoriasis, or colitis should be established. Clinical examination should include all joints, especially the spine and sacroiliac joints. Skin, nail, and eye examination should be documented.

This patient's diagnosis was enteropathic arthritis, with microcytosis due to gastrointestinal blood loss.

Six weeks later he was admitted with a 3-day history of severe abdominal pain associated with vomiting. He underwent laparotomy where he was found to have a 50cm segment of inflamed ileum proximal to the ileocaecal junction. Histology confirmed Crohn's disease (Figs 6.1–6.3).

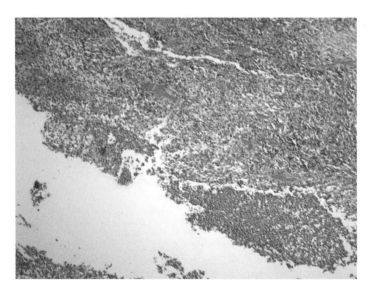

Fig. 6.1 (See also Plate 6) Linear fissuring ulcer formed by granulation tissue on either side, and containing neutrophils.

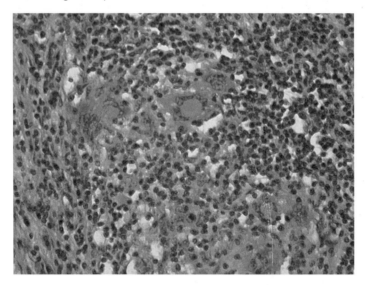

Fig. 6.2 (See also Plate 7) Granulomatous inflammation and giant cells.

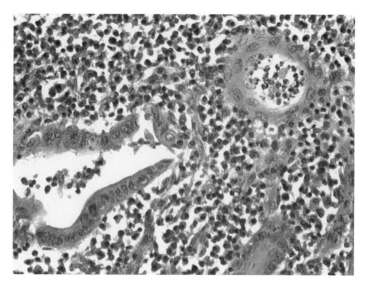

Fig. 6.3 (See also Plate 8) Distorted acutely inflamed colonic crypts (crypt abscesses).

Questions—Part 2

3. What are the treatment options?
4. How are his joint symptoms related to his Crohn's disease?

Answers

3. What are the treatment options?

First-line treatment for the joint disease is aspiration and intra-articular steroid injection to the affected joint(s).

The effect of drugs on the bowel needs to be considered in any treatment regime. Many patients are intolerant of NSAIDs, which can precipitate a flare of inflammatory GI symptoms. If joint symptoms do not settle with local steroid injections, sulfasalazine, methotrexate, or azathioprine are options. Anti-TNF treatments such as infliximab or adalimumab are currently used for severe Crohn's disease and enteropathic arthritis.

4. How are his joint symptoms related to his Crohn's disease?

The peripheral arthritis may be mono-, oligo-, or polyarticular. Some authorities suggest a classification into two groups. Type I is a large joint oligoarticular pattern, primarily affecting the knees and ankles, with self-limiting episodes often mirroring bowel activity. Type II is a symmetrical peripheral polyarthritis, involving both upper and lower limb. The clinical course of arthritis may run independently of the IBD, although in some patients a flare of arthritis can signal a flare of IBD. The prevalence and pattern of arthritis is similar in Crohn's disease and ulcerative colitis.

Approximately 20% of patients with IBD have inflammatory joint disease during the course of their illness. Symptoms are often episodic and variable, with 9% suffering inflammatory back pain, 2% having classical ankylosing spondyloarthritis (AS), and 5% having asymptomatic radiographic sacroiliitis.

Up to 5–10% of patients with spondyloarthritis have coexistent IBD. Between 30% and 60% of unselected spondyloarthritis patients have histological evidence of intestinal inflammation. Changes vary from an acute neutrophilic infiltrate of the lamina propria with intact architecture to more chronic changes with mononuclear cell infiltration of the lamina propria, aphthoid ulceration, and distortion of the villi and crypts. It is not yet known how frequently these changes progress to symptomatic IBD or whether treatment of arthritis alters the natural history of the gut changes.

Ankylosing spondylitis (AS) can precede IBD by many years and runs an independent clinical course. Peripheral arthritis, with associated dactylitis and enthesopathies, can again precede bowel symptoms. It is rarely erosive or deforming.

HLA B27 and CARD 15

Whilst over 90% of patients with isolated AS carry the HLA B27 gene, it is only carried by 70% of those with coexisting IBD and 20–50% of those with psoriatic spondylitis. Only 15% of individuals with IBD are HLA B27 positive. (HLA B27 positive patients are more likely to develop iritis, dactylitis, and sacroiliitis, but the association is much weaker than with AS).

Polymorphisms in the CARD 15 gene on chromosome 16 are associated with susceptibility to Crohn's disease, with homozygotes being at 38 times increased risk.

Thirty per cent to 46% of patients with Crohn's disease carry one of three mutations. The background population prevalence of these mutations is 20%. An increased rate of CARD 15 mutations is not found in isolated AS. However, there is an increased rate of CARD 15 mutation in those patients with a spondyloarthritis and histological evidence of gut inflammation, with 38% having a CARD 15 mutation.

Further reading

Brophy S, Pavy S, Lewis P, *et al.* (2001). Inflammatory eye, skin, and bowel disease in spondyloarthritis: genetic, phenotypic, and environmental factors. *J Rheumatol*; **28**: 2667–73.

Laukens D, Peeters H, Marichal D, *et al.* (2005). CARD15 gene polymorphisms in patients with spondyloarthropathies identify a specific phenotype previously related to Crohn's disease. *Ann Rheum Dis*; **64**: 930–5.

Palm Ø, Moum B, Jahnsen J, Gran JT (2001). The prevalence and incidence of peripheral arthritis in patients with inflammatory bowel disease, a prospective population-based study (the IBSEN study). *Rheumatology*; **40**: 1256–61.

Steer S, Jones H, Hibbert J, *et al.* (2003). Low back pain, sacroiliitis, and the relationship with HLA-B27 in Crohn's disease. *J Rheumatol*; **30**: 518–22.

Taurog JD (2006). Enteropathic arthritis. In: Fauci AS, Langford CA (eds). *Harrison's Rheumatology* (16th edn). New York: McGraw-Hill; 152–3.

Case 7

A 49-year-old Caucasian male presented with a 10-week history of bilateral swelling and stiffness of his MCP joints. His hands were stiff for 15 minutes every morning. He had a 10-year history of mechanical back pain and was on the waiting list for left hip replacement. He had had a right total knee replacement at age 40 years. He had previously been a high-level rugby player. Family history was unremarkable. On examination he had tender swelling of the second and third MCP joints of both hands. He had painless restriction of left ankle and subtalar joint movement.

Normal investigations included:

◆ FBC

◆ urea and electrolytes, liver function

◆ fasting glucose, calcium, uric acid

◆ ESR and CRP.

RF and ACCP antibody were negative.
Radiographs of the patient's hands, left ankle, and wrist are shown in Figs 7.1–7.4.

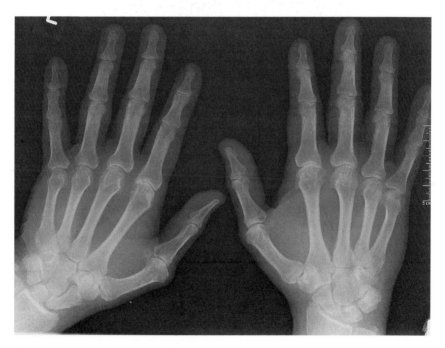

Fig. 7.1 Radiographs of patient's hands.

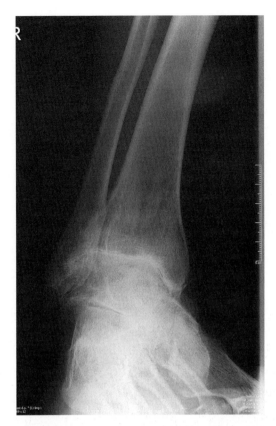

Fig. 7.2 Ankle X-ray showing severe osteoarthritic changes with almost complete loss of joint space, subchondral cysts, and sclerosis.

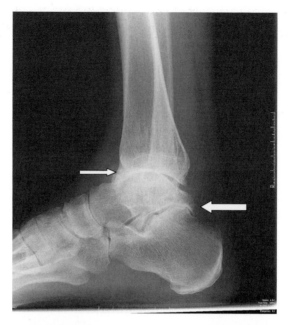

Fig. 7.3 Ankle X-ray showing severe osteoarthritic changes with almost complete loss of joint space, subchondral cysts and sclerosis, and large osteophytes (arrows).

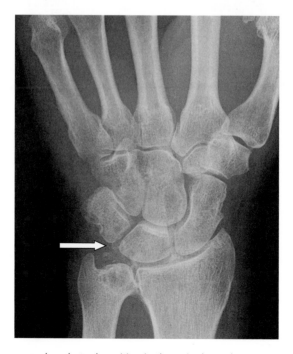

Fig. 7.4 Calcium pyrophosphate deposition in the wrist (arrow).

Questions

1. What is the differential diagnosis?
2. What specific laboratory investigations would you request?
3. What are the most likely diagnosis and clinical features of this condition?
4. What are the treatment strategies for the patient?
5. What are the implications for his relatives?

Answers

1. What is the differential diagnosis?

- Osteoarthritis (OA), especially secondary to trauma
- Early inflammatory arthritis
- Haemochromatosis
- Other causes of secondary chondrocalcinosis (hyperparathyroidism, hypomagnesaemia)
- Acromegaly.

The most likely diagnosis in a 49-year-old male presenting with mechanical hand pain and short-lived early morning stiffness is OA. The history of previous joint replacement and regular high-impact exercise may suggest accelerated OA secondary to trauma. However, the specific radiographic changes (Figs 7.1–7.4) prompt consideration of other underlying diagnoses.

Early inflammatory arthritis needs to be considered because of the MCP joint involvement and joint swelling. The short duration of early morning stiffness (less than 30 minutes), lack of an inflammatory response and absence of rheumatoid factor and ACCP antibodies make this diagnosis unlikely.

The presence of chondrocalcinosis on the radiographs means that the patient should be screened for diseases associated with calcium pyrophosphate deposition (CPPD) such as haemochromatosis, hyperparathyroidism, and hypomagnesaemia. His normal calcium is against a diagnosis of hyperparathyroidism.

Acromegaly (see p. 253) should be included in the differential diagnosis in the context of premature OA. Patients with acromegaly complain of non-specific arthralgia of the hands and large joints (shoulders, knees, spine, hips). Other clinical features (skin thickening and enlarged hands and feet, prominent forehead, and supra-orbital ridge) may help to diagnose the condition. Increased insulin like growth factor 1 will provide definite diagnosis. Radiographs in acromegaly may show widening of joint spaces due to cartilage overgrowth, or established OA in later stages.

2. What specific laboratory investigations would you request?

- Transferrin saturation (ratio of iron to total iron-binding capacity) is used for screening for haemochromatosis.
- If transferrin saturation is >50%, ferritin should be measured. In haemochromatosis, ferritin levels exceed 200 µg/L in pre-menopausal women and 300 µg/L in post-menopausal women and men.
- Both ferritin and transferrin act as acute phase reactants and levels may be high due to inflammatory disease elsewhere. Hence confirmation of diagnosis may require liver biopsy. Studies are exploring the use of CT and MRI to aid diagnosis.
- Genetic testing: haemochromatosis is an autosomal recessive disorder. It is due to mutations of the HFE gene located in the short arm of chromosome 6. HFE codes

a protein that acts in conjunction with β2-microglobulin to regulate intestinal iron absorption. The most common mutation is C282Y, and 90% of haemochromatosis patients are homozygous for HFE C282Y. Heterozygotes have increased iron stores but rarely develop clinical disease.

3. What are the most likely diagnosis and clinical features of this condition?

The most likely diagnosis is haemochromatosis.

Clues to the diagnosis are symptoms of accelerated osteoarthritis in a relatively young patient and hook osteophytes in the MCP joints. Repeated trauma related to his rugby playing career does not account for all these features. Patients with OA can experience morning stiffness, but not usually prolonged for more than 20 minutes.

Haemochromatosis is the most common autosomal recessive genetic disorder in people of Northern European extraction, particularly Celtic populations. One in 225 white Caucasian and 1 in 85 Irish are homozygous for the HFE C282Y gene. The prevalence of the disease is 30–60 in 10 000, with an estimated male-to-female ratio of 1.5:1. The disease presents in adult life, rarely before age 30, and men present on average 15 years before women. This is largely due to the protective effect of menstrual blood loss, although sex-specific differences in gene expression may be involved.

Excess intestinal absorption of iron with iron deposition in the parenchymal cells of many organs, including joints, liver, pituitary, heart, pancreas, and skin, leads to the clinical manifestation of the condition: arthritis (in ~40% of patients), cirrhosis, hypogonadism, cardiomyopathy, hypothyroidism (rare), diabetes mellitus, skin pigmentation, and bronze or slate-grey pigmentation. In the early stages patients may be asymptomatic or present non-specifically with lethargy, arthralgia, and loss of libido.

Haemochromatosis-associated arthritis affects the small joints of the hands (especially the second and third MCP joints) with hook-shaped osteophytes, as well as accelerating large-joint OA (hips, knees, ankles, and shoulders). Patients present with osteoarthritic symptoms between the ages of 30 and 60 but may present earlier. Haemochromatosis should always be suspected in young adults with OA even in the absence of other symptoms. Radiographs show subchondral sclerosis and cyst formation, space narrowing, and hook-like osteophytes. In 50% of cases there is evidence of calcium pyrophosphate deposition disease (CPDD), typically in the wrist, knee, intervertebral disc, and symphysis pubis, and patients may experience pseudo-gout attacks.

4. What are the treatment strategies for this patient?

Treatment strategies for this patient are to treat the iron overload, treat the arthritis, and assess for underlying organ damage, particularly liver disease.

The aims of treatment of iron overload are to rid the body of excess iron, maintain normal iron stores, and minimize dietary iron intake. Initially this requires once- or twice-weekly phlebotomy until serum ferritin is ≤20 µg/L. Subsequent maintenance phlebotomy (approximately four times per year) is needed to maintain this ferritin level.

General dietary advice includes minimizing oral iron intake, particularly red meat. Vitamin C increases intestinal iron absorption and supplements should be avoided. Alcohol also increases iron absorption; red wine has a high iron content and alcohol can accelerate liver damage. Therefore patients should avoid alcohol or limit intake to less than one unit per day.

Treatment of arthritis is symptomatic with analgesia, intra-articular steroid injections, orthotics, physiotherapy, exercise, and, in later stages, surgery. Any flares of associated chondrocalcinosis are treated symptomatically. Disease-modifying anti-rheumatic drugs (DMARDs) are unhelpful, and the arthropathy does not respond to iron removal.

The most important prognostic factor is the presence or absence of hepatic fibrosis or cirrhosis. Patients without liver disease have a normal life expectancy. The patient can have liver involvement with normal blood tests, and a liver biopsy is undertaken if the ferritin level is >1000 µg/L or the patient has abnormal LFTs. There are changes due to iron overload on both CT and MRI, but these cannot define fibrosis or cirrhosis. Patients with cirrhosis have a 200-fold increased risk of developing hepatocellular carcinoma and are screened by regular testing for α-fetoprotein levels plus liver ultrasound.

Pancreatic involvement is rare without cirrhosis, but patients with cirrhosis are at high risk of developing insulin-dependent diabetes. Hypogonadism from pituitary involvement is usually a late feature, although impotence is often an early feature. Cardiac involvement can lead to arrhythmias and cardiomyopathy. Patients can develop a slate-grey pigmentation which is caused by a combination of melanin and iron deposition. Excess mortality is usually from complications of cirrhosis, hepatocellular cancer, cardiomyopathy, or complications of diabetes.

Regular venepuncture leads to iron removal from tissues and prevents disease progression, particularly in early disease before irreversible parenchymal damage has occurred.

This patient's transferrin saturation was 60% and his serum ferritin level was 1450 µg/L. He was found to be homozygous for HFE C282Y. His alcohol intake was modest. He had regular venepuncture and he maintained normal liver function and low ferritin levels. He noted that his energy levels improved but his arthritis symptoms remained troublesome. He underwent a left total hip replacement, and took colchicine for episodes of wrist chondrocalcinosis flares.

5. What are the implications for his relatives?

First-degree relatives should be screened with transferrin saturation, serum ferritin, liver enzymes, and genotyping for the HFE mutation. Early diagnosis and treatment before organ damage occurs is associated with normal life expectancy.

The patient's only son was C282Y heterozygote with normal iron studies. His asymptomatic younger brother was also C282Y homozygous with significantly raised transferrin saturation and ferritin levels, and was referred for venepuncture treatment.

Further reading

Adams PC, Barton JC (2007). Haemochromatosis. *Lancet* 2007; **370**: 1855–60.

Cush J, Kavanaugh A, Stein CM (2005). *Rheumatology: Diagnosis and Therapeutics* (2nd edn). Philadelphia, PA: Lippincott–Williams & Wilkins.

Timms A, Sathananthan R, Bradbury L, Athanasou N, Wordsworth BP (2002). Genetic testing for haemochromatosis in patients with chondrocalcinosis. *Ann Rheum Dis*; **61**: 745–7.

Zhang W, Doherty M, Bardin T, *et al.* (2011). European League Against Rheumatism recommendations for calcium pyrophosphate deposition. Part I: Terminology and diagnosis. *Ann Rheum Dis*; **70**: 563–70.

Case 8

A 32-year-old man presented with a 6-month history of pain and swelling affecting both ankles and his left wrist. His past history included haemophilia A diagnosed at the age of 1 year after a bleeding episode from a cut lip. He had moderately severe disease with a baseline factor VIII level of 3%. At the age of 18, he was found to have acquired hepatitis C from contaminated blood products. At the age of 22 he was diagnosed with a large B-cell non-Hodgkin's lymphoma. He underwent treatment with chemotherapy and an autologous bone marrow transplant and was currently in remission.

On examination he had swelling of his wrist and both ankles and severe widespread plaque psoriasis. He had normal spinal movement.

Questions—Part 1

1. What is the differential diagnosis of his joint disease?
2. What further information would be helpful?

Answers

1. What is the differential diagnosis of his joint disease?

This is a case of oligoarthritis on a background of haemophilia, hepatitis C, psoriasis, and lymphoma. Leukaemia can present with joint swelling in the absence of haematological abnormalities, but arthritis is extremely rare as a presenting feature of lymphoma and is unlikely to be the underlying cause of his joint symptoms.

The differential diagnosis includes:

- haemophiliac arthropathy (HA)
- psoriatic arthritis
- viral arthritis
- reactive arthritis.

Haemophilia A is an X-linked recessive disorder of a deficiency or functional defect of coagulation factor VIII. Mild, moderate, and severe forms are defined by plasma coagulation factor levels. Joint disease affects 90% of people with severe haemophilia and occurs most commonly in the ankles, knees, and elbows. Coagulation levels of 5% or less are associated with recurrent haemarthrosis which can be spontaneous or due to trauma. Recurrent haemorrhage stimulates synovial hypertrophy and haemosiderin deposition, which in turn leads to further synovitis. The inflamed synovium is friable and prone to further haemorrhage. Subacute arthropathy follows repeated haemarthrosis affecting one or more target joints, especially ankles, knees, and elbows. Development of a target joint is indicated by a persistent boggy synovitis with chronic joint effusion and pain in the absence of recent haemorrhage. Muscle weakness and joint laxity increase the likelihood of further bleeding. The hyaline cartilage is eroded by both the inflamed synovium and direct toxic effects of iron deposition. A chronic HA may result, and may be severe with structural abnormalities, joint contractures due to fibrosis, and ankylosis.

HA was the most likely cause of this patient's recurrent ankle pain and swelling. However, the recent development of wrist swelling and the presence of psoriasis raised the possibility of psoriatic arthritis. A preceding history of bowel or genitourinary infection may indicate a reactive arthritis, and would be more likely to persist in patients who are positive for HLA B27. A further complicating feature of his case was his previous infection with hepatitis C.

Prior to 1992, hepatitis C and HIV were transmitted to many haemophiliacs from contaminated blood products, leading to chronic infection. Several viruses are associated with the development of inflammatory arthritis including the hepatitis viruses, HIV, and the parvovirus B19. The most common cause of arthritis in patients infected with hepatitis C is an unrelated inflammatory disease. Rarely, patients with chronic hepatitis C develop a directly related inflammatory arthritis. This is usually a symmetrical non-deforming non-erosive polyarthritis involving small joints, but may be a mono- or oligoarthritis.

Fewer than 5% of patients with hepatitis C develop mixed cryoglobulinaemia. This may present with intermittent polyarthralgia involving the hands and knees, immune-mediated purpura, neuropathy, membrano-proliferative glomerulone-phritis, and skin ulcers. The diagnosis is confirmed by the presence of type II or III cryoglobulins, low C4, and a positive rheumatoid factor.

2. What further information would be helpful?

i) Laboratory tests

FBC, viral serology for HIV, hepatitis B and E, and liver function tests. If further features of a mixed cryoglobulinaemia were present, it would be appropriate to measure cryoglobulins, renal function, rheumatoid factor, and urinalysis.

The patient had a normal FBC, CRP 52 g/dL, ALT 53 IU/L, and HIV serology was negative.

ii) Imaging

The early X-ray changes in HA include periarticular soft tissue swelling, bone dem-ineralization, and increased radiodensity of the thickened synovium due to haemo-siderin deposition. Where joint damage occurs in children, there may be Harris lines due to growth arrest and epiphysial widening. Some changes are specific to certain joints, for example squaring of the inferior border of the patella, tibiotalar slant, and enlargement of the proximal radial head. Established arthropathy is evi-dent by loss of joint space, subarticular sclerosis, osteophytes, cysts, joint disor-ganization, and bony ankylosis. However, plain films underestimate the degree of joint pathology. Ultrasound is useful in assessing soft tissue and synovial changes, and joint effusions in acute episodes.

MRI is the most sensitive examination for suspected HA, demonstrating syno-vial thickening, bleeding, and cartilage damage at an earlier stage than X-rays. A T_1-weighted sequence can be used to reveal early structural changes. A short T_1 inversion recovery (STIR) sequence will demonstrate bone oedema. Gradient echo sequences can be used to improve visualization of deoxyhaemoglobin in acute bleeds or haemosiderin deposition in chronic HA, and in this case would aid the differentiation between HA and psoriatic arthritis. However, when there is a sig-nificant amount of haemosiderin in a joint, visualization of joint structure may be impaired by susceptibility artefacts.

iii) Biopsy

Histological examination of a synovial biopsy may demonstrate a haemophiliac syn-ovitis with hypertrophy, monocytic infiltration, and deposition of haemosiderin.

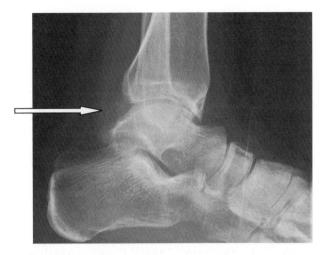

Fig. 8.1 Left ankle X-ray.

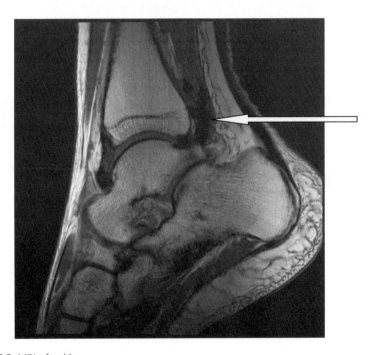

Fig. 8.2 MRI of ankle.

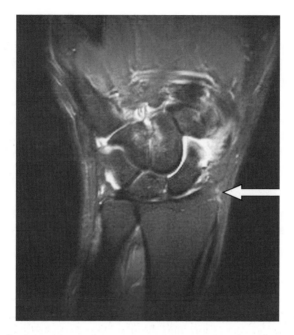

Fig. 8.3 MRI of wrist.

Questions—Part 2

3. Radiological images from this patient are shown in Figs 8.1–8.3. What do the arrows show and what is (are) the most likely diagnosis(es)?

4. How should his joint problems be managed? What is the role of factor VIII treatment in haemophilic arthropathy?

Answers

3. Radiological images from this patient are shown in Figs 8.1–8.3. What do the arrows show and what is (are) the most likely diagnosis(es)?

The ankle X-ray (Fig. 8.1) demonstrates haemosiderin deposition in the soft tissues. A susceptibility artefact caused by haemosiderin deposition along the tendon sheaths is shown by the arrow in Fig. 8.2 (ankle MRI). The wrist MRI (Fig. 8.3) shows evidence of synovitis with little haemosiderin deposition.

This patient was diagnosed with new-onset psoriatic arthritis on a background of HA.

4. How should his joint problems be managed? What is the role of factor VIII treatment in haemophilic arthropathy?

Management of an acute haemarthrosis in haemophilia includes 48 hours of synthetic factor VIII, and local measures to manage the joint swelling and pain (ice packs, analgesia, and physiotherapy). The development of a 'boggy synovitis' indicates potential irreversible joint damage and preventative treatment may be started with secondary prophylaxis using factor VIII replacement three times weekly for 6–8 weeks to controlling bleeding. Muscle strength is improved with physiotherapy. NSAIDs should be used with caution, and there is no benefit from DMARDs. Intra-articular steroids can produce short-term benefit.

This patient was administered factor VIII injections at the onset of ankle swelling but did not respond to treatment. He was diagnosed with psoriatic arthritis on the basis of psoriasis, raised inflammatory markers, and MRI evidence of wrist synovitis without haemosiderin. He was treated with intra-articular joint injections under factor VIII prophylaxis and physiotherapy.

In view of his history of hepatitis C, his treatment with medications such as methotrexate and subsequently leflunomide was planned in collaboration with a hepatologist. In patients without advanced liver disease and with stable liver function, these medications can be used safely with close monitoring. Studies looking at the safety of anti-TNF agents in patients with chronic hepatitis C are under way. The patient's joints improved on methotrexate but, unusually, his psoriasis deteriorated. Treatment was changed to leflunomide which improved both psoriasis and joint symptoms.

Primary prophylaxis by regular long-term administration of clotting factor concentrate is the first choice of treatment in children with severe haemophilia. This is implemented either before the age of 2 years and prior to any joint bleeding, or after no more than one joint bleed. The Joint Outcome Study in 2007 was the first randomized controlled trial of prophylaxis versus on-demand treatment. It showed an 85% reduction in the risk of joint damage by MRI assessment in children on prophylaxis (25 IU/kg every other day) compared with those using intensive on-demand treatments.

In some patients, a secondary prophylaxis regimen is prescribed for short periods to reduce the frequency of bleeds in target joints. Published evidence on the benefits of long-term secondary prophylaxis in young adult haemophiliacs has been from small retrospective studies. They show that severe haemophiliac adults switching from on-demand to secondary prophylaxis used more concentrate but had fewer joint bleeds. Secondary prophylaxis has not yet been shown to slow the progression of HA in patients with established joint damage. Various radiological scoring systems have been developed to monitor disease progression by MRI and are important in measuring response to prophylactic factor VIII treatment.

Further reading

Coppola A, Di Capua M, Simone CD (2008). Primary prophylaxis in children with haemophilia. *Blood Transfus*; **6**(Suppl 2): s4–11.

Jelbert A, Vaidya S, Fotiadis N (2009). Imaging and staging of haemophilic arthropathy. *Clin Radiol*; **64**: 1119–28.

Tagliaferri A, De Perna C, Rivolta GF (2008). Secondary prophylaxis in adolescents and adult haemophiliacs. *Blood Transfus*; **6**(Suppl 2): s17–20.

Vassilopoulos D, Calabrese LH (2008). Virally associated arthritis 2008: clinical, epidemiologic, and pathophysiologic considerations. *Arthritis Res Ther*; **10**: 215.

Case 9

A 30-year-old female with a 10-year history of systemic lupus erythematosus (SLE) was reviewed in clinic. She had recently married and was keen to start a family. At diagnosis she had presented with a photosensitive rash, fleeting arthralgia, migraine, depression, and proteinuria. A renal biopsy had confirmed membranous glomerulonephritis, consistent with class V lupus nephritis. She was initially treated with prednisolone and azathioprine, but ongoing active renal disease necessitated escalation to cyclophosphamide and subsequent maintenance therapy with mycophenolate mofetil 1g twice daily.

Examination was normal, including a blood pressure of 120/80 mmHg. Dipstick urinalysis was normal.

Questions—Part 1

1. How would you assess her disease activity? What other tests would you consider in preparation for pregnancy?

2. What pre-conception counselling would you provide with regard to the following?

   i. Medication and contraception.

   ii. Renal disease.

   iii. Pregnancy-related risks? What additional monitoring may be required during pregnancy?

Answers

1. How would you assess her disease activity? What other tests would you consider in preparation for pregnancy?

Pregnancy outcome is better if conception occurs during a period of remission, or 6 months after control of a flare or a change in maintenance therapy.

Disease activity in SLE can be assessed using the SLE Disease Activity Index, a global disease activity score (DAS) validated against experienced clinical judgement used to quantify organ involvement and guide therapeutic management.

Pre-conception all patients with SLE should be screened for a lupus anticoagulant, antiphospholipid, and anti-Ro and anti-La antibodies. Anticoagulants including aspirin and heparin have been shown to improve pregnancy outcome in women with antiphospholipid syndrome (APS) (see p. 75). Ds DNA, anti-Ro antibodies, and anti-La antibodies may result in neonatal lupus which requires further monitoring (see Answer 2).

2. What pre-conception counselling would you provide with regard to the following?

 i. Medication and contraception.

 ii. Renal disease.

 iii. Pregnancy-related risks. What additional monitoring may be required during pregnancy?

 i. Patients taking teratogenic medications should be advised regarding contraception, avoiding oestrogen-containing preparations due to the risk of flare. Animal studies suggest that mycophenolate mofetil is associated with an increase in congenital malformations and should be avoided in pregnancy. It is standard practice to switch to azathioprine and hydroxychloroquine, as was done in this case, which are considered safe in pregnancy.

 ii. There is a risk of deterioration in renal function due to the change in medication or as a result of pregnancy. The risk is higher with pre-existing hypertension, proteinuria (>1 g/24h), or high baseline serum creatinine (>125 µmol/L).

 iii. Lupus itself does not usually affect fertility, but NSAIDs, previous cyclophosphamide treatment, and ongoing disease activity may prevent conception. There are increased risks of early miscarriage, intra-uterine fetal death, pre-eclampsia, intra-uterine growth retardation, and pre-term delivery. Pregnancy may increase the risk of flare both antenatally and in the puerperium. Patients with active lupus, particularly if nephrotic, are at increased risk of venous thromboembolism (VTE) in pregnancy. Therefore it is imperative that a detailed history is taken of previous history of clots or other risk factors, and thromboprophylaxis should be considered. Women with APS are at increased risk of VTE and fetal loss, and low-dose aspirin and low molecular weight heparin are recommended throughout pregnancy and 6 weeks post-natally. Such patients should be managed under collaborative care of obstetrics and haematology.

Increased maternal and fetal surveillance is required during pregnancy, particularly in women with hypertension, renal disease, APS, and Ro antibodies. Ro antibodies are associated with congenital heart block in 1–2% of cases; early cardiac fetal monitoring is important in detecting this as it can result in intra-uterine death. Ro and La antibodies can cross the placenta and 5% of babies may suffer a neonatal lupus syndrome which is transient.

She conceived 8 months later and was initially well, but at 21 weeks' gestation was noted to have deteriorating renal function and hypertension (BP 170/110 mmHg). Investigations showed:

- urea 18 mmol/L
- creatinine 171 μmol/L
- albumin 16 g/dL
- urinary protein 10 g/24 h.

Questions—Part 2

3. There are two main causes of this presentation, what further investigations would you request in order to differentiate between the two?

Answer

3. There are two main causes of this presentation. What further investigations would you request in order to differentiate between the two?

Deteriorating renal function, hypertension, and proteinuria suggest a flare of her lupus nephritis, pre-eclampsia, or both. These conditions are potentially life-threatening to both mother and baby. The features distinguishing a lupus flare and pre-eclampsia are shown in Table 9.1.

Steroids are first-line therapy for lupus flare during pregnancy. Prednisolone is inactivated by placental 11 β-hydroxysteroid dehydrogenase 2 so that only 10% of the active drug reaches the fetus. High-dose steroids increase the risk of maternal gestational diabetes, hypertension, infection, and osteoporosis. Other immuno-suppressive agents that are considered to be safe in pregnancy include azathioprine, hydroxychloroquine, ciclosporin, tacrolimus, and intravenous immunoglobulin. There are few data for the use of biological agents such as anti-TNF therapy, but so far there is no suggestion of adverse maternal or fetal outcome. In rare severe cases, cyclophosphamide has been used in pregnancy.

Table 9.1 Features distinguishing a lupus flare from pre-eclampsia

	Lupus flare	Pre-eclampsia
Hypertension	Yes	Yes
Urine analysis	Proteinuria	Red cell casts and proteinuria
Platelet count	Low	Low
Abnormal LFTs	Unusual	Common
Creatinine	Raised	Raised
Serology	Raised dsDNA and low C3/C4	Normal
Uric acid	Normal	High

Further reading

Bombardier C, Gladman DD, Urowitz MB, Caron D, Chang CH (1992). Derivation of the SLEDAI. A disease activity index for lupus patients. The Committee on Prognosis Studies in SLE. *Arthritis Rheum*; **35**: 630–40.

Mackillop LH, Germain SJ, Nelson-Piercy C (2007). Systemic lupus erythematosus. *BMJ*; **335**: 933–6.

Case 10

A 73-year-old woman was admitted to the trauma ward with a fractured neck of femur after falling from her chair. Despite fixation surgery with a good technical result, her rehabilitation was slow and she complained of generalized muscle aches. Her past medical history was unremarkable apart from anaemia, treated with three-monthly B_{12} injections.

Twelve months prior to her fall, she had developed severe pain and stiffness affecting both shoulders, unresponsive to steroid, with limited movement preventing her from playing lawn bowls. The shoulder pain did not resolve after steroid injections into her shoulders. Furthermore, she was not able to return to her bowls as she developed reduced grip strength and numbness of her right thumb and index finger.

She had difficulty getting out of bed in the morning and would tend to sit in her chair, by her heater, for most of the day as she found it difficult to stand up because of weakness in her thighs. Her daughter was worried as her mother was becoming increasingly withdrawn and sedentary.

Questions

1. Based on the history, which aspects of the musculoskeletal and neurological systems have been affected?
2. What is the most likely unifying diagnosis?
3. Which rheumatological and other conditions have been associated with an autoimmune cause for this underlying diagnosis?
4. What factors may have contributed to her risk of fracture?

Answers

1. Based on the history, which aspects of the musculoskeletal and neurological systems have been affected?

The clinical features of this case suggest:

- proximal myopathy
- carpal tunnel syndrome
- bilateral shoulder adhesive capsulitis
- fragility fracture.

2. What is the most likely unifying diagnosis?

The most likely unifying diagnosis is hypothyroidism, which can affect up to 14% of the elderly population. Patients often present with myalgia, proximal muscle weakness, which may be associated with a mild elevation in CK, and arthralgia. This patient had symptoms of a proximal myopathy with quadriceps weakness. Nerve-entrapment syndromes are common, with carpal tunnel syndrome occurring in 30% of patients with hypothyroidism in one series. Adhesive capsulitis was reported in 11% of patients with thyroid disease, including those with hyperthyroid, hypothyroid, and euthyroid states. This is higher than the reported prevalence of primary idiopathic adhesive capsulitis in the general population of 2–3%.

Lethargy, weight gain, cold intolerance, depression, poor memory, change in appearance, dry hair, and dry skin are other features which should be sought in the history. Mild haemolysis can also occur with hypothyroidism, which would contribute further to this woman's anaemia and lethargy.

3. Which rheumatological and other conditions have been associated with an autoimmune cause for this underlying diagnosis?

Chronic autoimmune thyroiditis, characterized by diffuse lymphocytic infiltration of the thyroid gland, presence of antithyroid antibodies in the serum and frequently thyroid dysfunction, has been associated with a variety of rheumatic manifestations. In addition to the features attributed to hypothyroidism, described above, there are a collection of autoimmune rheumatic diseases which may overlap with autoimmune thyroid disease *per se*.

Autoimmune thyroid disease occurs in more than one-third of patients with primary Sjögren's syndrome, and Sjögren's syndrome is present with similar frequency in autoimmune thyroid disease. Therefore screening should be conducted in these groups of patients. Recent studies have also demonstrated a high frequency of autoimmune thyroid disease in patients with rheumatoid arthritis (RA), as well as in their families. The overlap in symptoms, including lethargy and muscle and joint pains, highlights the need to screen RA patients.

Other rheumatological conditions with a less clear link include SLE, scleroderma, and polymyalgia rheumatica (PMR). Muscle symptoms including pain, weakness, and cramps, sometimes associated with raised creatine kinase (CK) may be seen with hypothyroidism. However, clinical and biochemical features of muscle dysfunction can also occur in the context of subclinical hypothyroidism. Patients with euthyroid autoimmune thyroid disease have also been found to demonstrate electron microscopic capillary abnormalities and macrophage, lymphocytic, and mast cell infiltration of skeletal muscle.

4. What factors may have contributed to her risk of fracture?

Fracture risk is multifactorial in patients with hypothyroidism. Risk of falling is increased by proximal muscle weakness, arthralgia, peripheral sensorimotor neuropathy, bradycardia, heart failure, slowness of thought, and poor attention.

Fragility fractures are seen in both hypothyroidism and hyperthyroidism. Hyperthyroidism is associated with increased bone resorption, reduced bone mineral density (BMD), and so increased fracture. Hypothyroidism results in a reduction in osteoblastic and osteoclastic activity, leading to prolongation of the remodelling cycle with reduced bone turnover. Although BMD subsequently tends to be higher than normal in patients with hypothyroidism, fracture risk remains increased. Reduced bone quality, rather than dual-energy X-ray absorptiometry (DEXA) score, may explain this link. It is still unclear whether thyroxine therapy itself also has a deleterious effect on bone.

Further reading

McLean RM, Podell DN (1995). Bone and joint manifestations of hypothyroidism. *Semin Arthritis Rheum*; **24**: 282–90.

Punzi L, Betterle C (2004). Chronic autoimmune thyroiditis and rheumatic manifestations. *Joint Bone Spine*; **71**: 275–83.

Case 11

A 26-year-old female graduate student was admitted to the acute admissions unit with a 12-hour history of rapid-onset fever, left-sided pleuritic chest pain, and a swollen left knee. There was no shortness of breath or haemoptysis. Her knee was hot, red, and swollen, and she was unable to weight bear. She had small tender red swellings over the dorsum of her right foot.

She had recently returned from a holiday in Gibraltar where she had visited her grandparents. She had no history of insect bite, infection, or excessive sun exposure. She was previously healthy, apart from a recurrent febrile tonsillitis throughout childhood, severe dysmenorrhoea, and appendectomy aged 17. She was married and was under investigation for primary infertility. She has no past or family history of arthritis, enthesitis, iritis, arthritis, photosensitive rash, mouth ulcers, or Raynaud's phenomenon.

On examination her temperature was 40°C, pulse 100 beats/min, BP 130/80 mmHg, respiratory rate 15 breaths/min, chest clear to auscultation. She had a tense effusion around her left knee and a skin rash with three red, raised, tender, well-demarcated flat lesions 2 cm in diameter over the dorsum of her right foot. She had no other joint swelling, and her skin and nails were otherwise normal.

She was admitted and 30 mL of murky fluid was aspirated from her knee. She was started on intravenous flucloxacillin. Six hours after the infusion had started the chest pain resolved completely. The intravenous antibiotics were continued for 48 hours. The knee remained swollen and red for a further 3 days. The swelling gradually resolved over the course of the next 3 weeks.

Investigations showed the following:

- Hb 12.6 g/dL; WCC 11.5 × 10⁹/L; neutrophils 4.3 × 10⁹/L; platelets 448 × 10⁹/L
- Blood film normal
- Blood cultures: no growth on prolonged culture
- Throat swab: no growth
- LFTs normal
- GFR normal
- CXR clear
- ECG normal
- ANA negative; RF negative; ANCA negative; complement levels normal
- ASOT <200 units/mL
- CRP 70 mg/L
- Dipstick urinalysis: + protein; MSU no growth
- Joint aspirate: >100 WCC/hpf. No other cells, organisms, or crystals. No growth on prolonged culture.

Questions

1. What is the differential diagnosis?
2. What is the likely diagnosis?
3. How is the diagnosis is usually made?
4. What is the treatment and prognosis?

Answers

1. What is the differential diagnosis

There is a wide differential diagnosis in this woman:

- septic arthritis
- SLE
- acute rheumatic fever
- reactive arthritis
- adult Still's disease
- acute sarcoidosis
- periodic fever syndrome.

Septic arthritis is the most important diagnosis to exclude, and giving parenteral flucloxacillin (plus penicillin depending on local antibiotic policy) until cultures are negative is standard practice.

The negative auto-antibody screen excludes SLE and makes other connective tissue diseases unlikely.

Patients with acute sarcoidosis usually present with periarthritis rather than arthritis, erythema nodosum and have hilar lymphadenopathy on CXR, and erythema nodosum skin lesions. In this patient the CXR, arthritis rather than periarthritis, and flat skin lesions were all against the diagnosis of acute sarcoid.

Reactive arthritis rarely presents with pleuritic chest pain. Associated rashes are palmo-plantar pustulosis or keratoderma blennorrhagica on the soles and palms rather than on the dorsum of the feet.

Acute rheumatic fever is an important diagnosis to exclude, particularly with a past history of recurrent childhood tonsillitis. The rash of acute rheumatic fever, erythema marginatum, classically affects the trunk and upper limbs and not the feet. The lack of laboratory evidence for streptococcal infection makes the diagnosis unlikely.

It is important to re-evaluate the previous childhood febrile episodes. Her mother and maternal grandparents were from Gibraltar and of Jewish descent. Her father was Turkish and she had been raised in the UK.

Her childhood febrile tonsillitis episodes usually started dramatically, with high fevers developing during the course of a few hours. The episodes lasted up to 3 days and were sometimes associated with abdominal pain and aching wrists. She was well between attacks.

Her appendectomy occurred during one of these episodes, when the abdominal pain worsened rather than improved overnight. She was told that the appendix was normal.

She was used to having attacks of lesser fevers before her periods, which were always painful and associated initially with constipation, and then diarrhoea.

She and her husband had been trying to conceive for a year and were just considering referral for fertility investigations.

2. What is the likely diagnosis?

A likely diagnosis is familial Mediterranean fever (FMF) which is one of the auto-inflammatory syndromes.

The recurrent febrile episodes in childhood can be misdiagnosed as tonsillitis. The severe dysmenorrhoea and appendectomy probably represented mild episodes of abdominal serositis.

The presenting episode was more severe, with symptoms of fever, pleurisy, cutaneous lesions, and monoarthritis. The classical skin lesions are sharply bordered, hot, tender erysipelas-like plaques 10–35 mm in diameter occurring on the extensor surface of the ankle or the dorsum of the foot, appearing with the rapidly rising fever. The dipstick proteinuria is important to follow as it may suggest early amyloidosis.

3. How is the diagnosis usually made?

The diagnosis can be made clinically on the basis of typical attacks in an individual from the appropriate ethnic population.

FMF characteristically affects people descended from Sephardic (Spanish from North Africa) Jews, and is less common amongst East European Jews, Anatolian Turks, Arabs, Armenians, and other Mediterranean groups. Intermarriage and migration means that the condition can occur sporadically in most populations.

Tel Hashomer criteria for the diagnosis of familial Mediterranean fever

◆ Major:
  • recurrent febrile episodes accompanied by peritonitis, synovitis, or pleuritis
  • amyloidosis of amyloid A type without predisposing disease
  • favourable response to colchicine.
◆ Minor:
  • recurrent febrile episodes
  • erysipelas-like erythema
  • FMF in a first-degree relative.
◆ Definitive diagnosis—two major or one major and two minor.
◆ Probable diagnosis—one major and one minor.

Specificity in a Jewish population is >95%.

Gene testing

This is an autosomal recessive condition. Genetic screening is now possible for common mutations in the FMF gene. The MEFV gene is located on the short arm of chromosome 16p13.3. It is a 10-exon gene encoding pyrin (a 781 amino acid protein). Pyrin is expressed in myeloid cells and is believed to regulate inflammation via apoptosis.There are four common missense or nonsense mutations which produce different clinical patterns.

Testing for amyloid

In this patient, the presence of proteinuria, if persistent, suggests AA amyloidosis. The gold standard for diagnosis is the presence of biopsy-proven amyloid deposits. The biopsy sites used are abdominal fat aspiration (safe outpatient test, 55–75% sensitive), rectal biopsy (uncomfortable, risk of rectal bleeding, 75–85% sensitive), and liver or kidney biopsy (risk of life-threatening bleed from vascular amyloid deposits, 99% sensitive).

Biopsy is becoming superseded by total body scintigraphy using radiolabelled serum amyloid protein (SAP). This is a sensitive non-invasive technique that locates and quantifies amyloid deposits throughout the body. Affected organs are highlighted and the test can be repeated to follow the effects of treatment and progress.

4. What is the treatment and prognosis?

Acute attacks are self-limiting and require simple analgesia and NSAIDs. Attacks occur at irregular intervals with no clear precipitating cause.

Severe abdominal pain is the first presentation in 70% of cases and is the most frequent manifestation, occurring in 90% of patients. Symptoms and signs can resemble an acute abdomen and appendectomy is often undertaken (with normal histology). Attacks reach a peak within a few hours and start to abate after 6–12 hours. Most patients return to normal within 24–48 hours.

Fertility is sometimes impaired in women because pelvic adhesions can develop after frequent abdominal attacks. Treatment with colchicine lessens the frequency of attacks, the development of adhesions, and the rate of early miscarriage.

Arthritis affects 75% of patients, and is the second most common presentation. Classically, patients present with painful sterile monoarthritis of a hip or knee. Most resolve over 48–72 hours and NSAIDs plus colchicine are usually sufficient to control symptoms whilst attacks settle. Five per cent develop a chronic destructive arthritis which can lead to aseptic necrosis and require joint arthroplasty.

Acute febrile pleurisy occurs in 45% of patients. Although painful, it is benign and resolves within 48 hours with no significant sequelae.

The most serious long-term complication is AA amyloidosis with renal failure. The risk of developing AA amyloidosis increases if there is a family history of amyloidosis and varies between genetic mutations, with the M694V mutation having the highest risk.

Treatment is with colchicine (1–2 mg/day) which reduces the duration of acute attacks, prevents further acute inflammatory attacks, and prevents the long-term development of amyloidosis. Colchicine also decreases the rate of progression of established amyloid.

Colchicine is usually well tolerated; the most common side effects are diarrhoea and nausea which patients adjust to. Compliance can be difficult, particularly with teenagers. However, even short breaks from treatment can result in flare of disease and development of AA amyloid. Pregnancy is usually associated with remission of symptoms. However, it is usually recommended that colchicine treatment is continued during pregnancy, as the flares of disease can lead to miscarriage.

Long-term follow-up is needed with regular urinalysis and renal function testing to detect early amyloid.

Patients with amyloidosis need careful hypertensive control and usually progress to renal failure and transplantation in their fifties.

Prior to colchicine therapy, amyloidosis caused by FMF was universally fatal by the early forties.

Corticosteroids are generally ineffective during acute attacks and in preventing development of amyloidosis.

Approximately 10% of FMF patients are resistant or non-responsive to colchicine treatment. There are early reports that the IL-1 receptor antagonist anakinra is effective in treating colchicine-resistant cases.

Further reading

Diav-Citrin O, Shechtman S, Schwartz V, *et al.* (2010). Pregnancy outcome after *in utero* exposure to colchicine. *Am J Obstet Gynecol*; **203**: 144.

Livneh A, Langevitz P, Zemer D, *et al.* (1997). Criteria for the diagnosis of familial Mediterranean fever. *Arthritis Rheum*; **40**: 1879–85.

Yao Q, Furst D (2008). Autoinflammatory diseases: an update of clinical and genetic aspects. *Rheumatology*; **47**: 946–51.

Zemer D, Pras M, Sohar E, Modan B, Cabili S, Gafni J (1986). Colchicine in the prevention and treatment of amyloidosis of familial Mediterranean fever. *N Engl J Med*; **314**: 1001–5.

Case 12

A teenager presented to her GP concerned about her appearance as she was teased at school. She was the tallest in her class and thinner than her peer group. She had disproportionately long limbs and a concave chest wall. Clinical examination revealed a systolic murmur.

Questions

1. What is the differential diagnosis?
2. What is Marfan's syndrome?
3. Which gene is involved and what is the recommended genetic screening?
4. What are the long-term complications of Marfan's syndrome?
5. What advice regarding sport should be given to a patient with Marfan's syndrome?

Answers

1. What is the differential diagnosis?

The differential diagnosis is:

- constitutional tall stature
- Marfanoid habitus
- Marfan's syndrome
- pituitary hypersecretion of growth hormone (GH) (gigantism)
- Ehlers–Danlos syndrome
- homocystinuria
- congenital contractural arachnodactyly.

If the patient's height is greater than the 95th percentile, it should be compared with her expected height which can be calculated from parental height and may be normal. She may have a Marfanoid habitus which might be associated with hyper-mobility but not with disease manifestations.

Congenital contractural arachnodactyly is an autosomal dominant condition caused by mutations in the FBN2 gene and results in a tall slender habitus with long fingers, crumpled ears, and arm span exceeding height, but with normal eyes and aorta. Homocystinuria may present with skeletal features similar to Marfan's syndrome and a downward lens dislocation. This is a recessively inherited inborn error of amino acid metabolism due to a deficiency of cystathionine β-synthetase. Patients have a positive urine cyanide–nitroprusside test to detect homocysteine.

2. What is Marfan's syndrome?

Marfan's syndrome is a multisystem disorder of connective tissue which is generally inherited as an autosomal dominant condition but occurs after sporadic mutation in 25% of cases. It is one of the most common single-gene malformation syndromes with a prevalence of 1 in 5000–10 000. Isolated clinical features are common; many clinicians will encounter potential cases, and diagnostic accuracy is relevant not only for the patient but also for family members.

It is characterized by arachnodactyly, tall stature, pectus deformities of the chest, facial and eye abnormalities, and mandibular hypoplasia. There are no unique characteristics but more than 35 clinical features may be variably associated.

The diagnosis is based on the Ghent criteria which include clinical features from the skeletal, ocular, cardiovascular, and pulmonary systems, the dura, and the skin, and family or genetic history. A diagnosis of Marfan's syndrome requires the presence of a major criterion in two systems and involvement of a third.

Major criteria

- Skeletal:
  - pectus carinatum or pectus excavatum requiring surgery
  - upper to lower segment ratio <0.86, or span to height ratio >1.05
  - wrist and thumb signs

- scoliosis >20°
- reduced elbow extension <170°
- pes planus
- protrusio acetabulae.

◆ Dura:
  - lumbosacral dural ectasia.

◆ Cardiovascular:
  - dilatation of the aortic root
  - dissection of the ascending aorta.

◆ Ocular:
  - ectopia lentis.

◆ Genetic:
  - first-degree relative meets criteria independently
  - presence of FBN-1 mutation.

Minor criteria

The minor criteria define involvement of a particular organ system and can be included in the diagnosis of Marfan's syndrome if major criteria are also present. They include pectus excavatum of moderate severity, joint hypermobility, high arched palate, dental crowding, characteristic facies, flat cornea, hypoplastic iris, mitral valve prolapse, calcified mitral annulus, dilatation of the pulmonary artery, spontaneous pneumothorax, apical blebs, striae atrophicae, and recurrent or incisional hernia.

3. Which gene is involved and what is the recommended genetic screening?

Marfan's syndrome is caused by mutations in a single fibrillin gene (FBN1) on chromosome 15. Fibrillin is a glycoprotein produced by fibroblasts and aggregates in the extracellular matrix, forming the meshwork on which elastin is deposited. Elastin fibres are abundant in the aorta, ligaments, and the ciliary zonules of the lens, and these areas are characteristically affected in the condition. A transgenic mouse has been created to carry a single copy of a mutant fibrillin-1 gene, and demonstrates many features of Marfan's syndrome.

Fibrillin-1 indirectly binds an inactive form of transforming growth factor-β (TGF-β). A mechanism of disease has been suggested whereby reduced levels of fibrillin-1 result in a rise in TGF-β resulting in an inflammatory reaction and release of elastin degrading proteases.

Genetic screening may be useful in defining new mutations. The risks to other family members are different depending on whether the mutation is inherited or spontaneous, and family members sharing an identical mutation may show great clinical variety. It is important to make a clear diagnosis of Marfan's syndrome as it is a cause of preventable sudden death in young adults. Patients should be included in a screening programme for cardiovascular, ophthalmological, and musculoskeletal complications.

4. What are the long-term complications of Marfan's syndrome?

The main cardiovascular complications are aortic root enlargement, mitral valve prolapse, and arrhythmias. Routine care includes annual echocardiography and an electrocardiogram. Risk factors for aortic dissection include an aortic diameter >5 cm, aortic dilatation extending beyond the sinus of Valsalva, a rapid rate of aortic root dilatation, or a family history of aortic dissection. Aggressive management of aortic root dilatation with β-blockers reduces the risk of dissection. Patients are referred for prophylactic aortic root surgery when the diameter at the sinus of Valsalva exceeds 5.5 cm in an adult or 5 cm in a child. Pregnant women with Marfan's syndrome are at increased risk of aortic dissection when the aortic root diameter is ≥4 cm in the presence of aortic dilatation.

A number of ophthalmological complications are associated with Marfan's syndrome. Approximately 60% have ectopia lentis which is managed with miotic drugs to constrict the pupil and refractive lenses. Patients frequently have strabismus, requiring treatment to prevent amblyopia. There is an increased risk of retinal detachment as the globe is elongated.

Kyphosis and scoliosis may develop during childhood. A scoliosis beyond 40° may contribute to restrictive lung disease, resulting in cor pulmonale, and require corrective surgery. Pectus excavatum may require surgery in early adulthood as the reduced spinal–sternum diameter may lead to cardiac complications. Pectus carinatum rarely causes medical complications but may be repaired for cosmetic reasons.

Figure 12.1 shows an MRI of a marked thoracolumbar scoliosis in Marfan's syndrome, convex to the right.

Dural ectasia is a dilation of the dural sac, usually at the L5–S1 level of the spine (Fig. 12.2) and can occur in two-thirds of adults with Marfan's syndrome. It typically presents with unremitting headache or spinal pain and may cause peripheral neurological symptoms due to nerve root pressure, such as referred pain, weakness, or loss of bladder control.

It may be treated conservatively with gabapentin, physiotherapy, and hydrotherapy, but may require neurosurgical repair of the dura for symptomatic relief.

5. What advice regarding sport should be given to a patient with Marfan's syndrome?

Low to moderate degrees of activity are advised for patients with Marfan's syndrome depending on the presence of risk factors, and a reduction of physical and haemodynamic stress may be advised for those with cardiopulmonary or ophthalmological disease. Patients are advised about the dangers associated with some sports and to avoid those that involve blows to the head and eye such as boxing and some racquet sports. Contact sports and high diving should be avoided because of the risks of aortic dissection and lens dislocation. Patients who have undergone aortic root or valve replacements may need further caution, particularly if receiving anticoagulation. Diving should be avoided because of the risk of spontaneous pneumothorax.

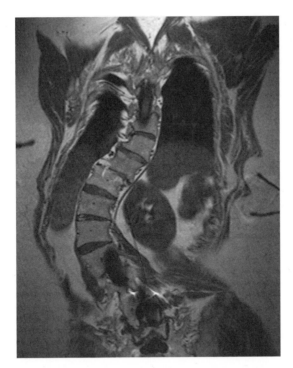

Fig. 12.1 T$_1$-weighted MRI scan of the spine in a patient with Marfan's syndrome.

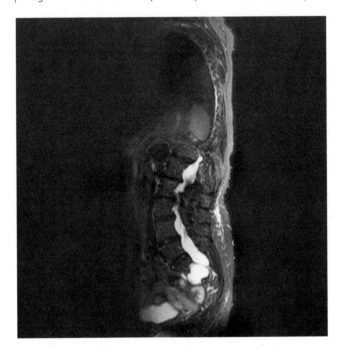

Fig. 12.2 Dural ectasia with a large cystic cerebrospinal fluid (CSF) out-pouching extending through the left S2 exit foramen. (Note: this is not the same patient as in Fig. 12.1).

Follow-up

This patient developed dyspnoea and bilateral pedal oedema due to mitral valve prolapse when she was 25 years old and underwent a 33 mm Bjork–Shiley tilting mitral valve replacement. Regular echocardiograms demonstrated aortic root dilatation of 6 cm at the age of 30 years and she underwent an aortic root replacement.

Further reading

de Paepe A, Devereux RB, Dietz HC, Hennekam RC, Pyeritz RE (1996). Revised diagnostic criteria for the Marfan syndrome. *Am J Med Genet*; **62**: 417–26.

Ho NCY, Tran JR, Bektas A (2005). Marfan's syndrome. *Lancet*; **366**: 1978–81.

Summers KM, Wes JA, Peterson MM, Stark D, McGill JJ, West MJ (2006). Challenges in the diagnosis of Marfan syndrome. *Med J Aust*; **184**: 627–31.

Case 13

A 12-year-old girl presented with a 4-week history of involuntary choreiform movements when walking, initially affecting her right arm, progressing to involve her left arm, legs, and subsequently her face, head, and trunk. It interfered with dressing and feeding herself. She had dysphasia and was noted to have easy bruising. There was no past medical history, but her paternal grandmother had Sydenham's chorea as a child. She had normal cardiovascular, respiratory, and abdominal examinations, and normal eye movements and fundoscopy. She had small widespread bruises and a mottled rash on her legs (Fig. 13.1). A full blood count showed her to have a thrombocytopenia with platelets of 58×10^9/L.

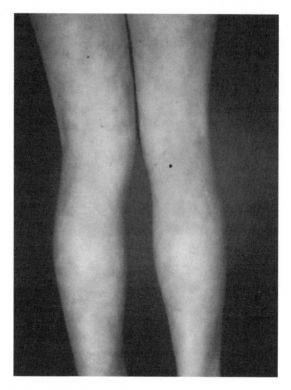

Fig. 13.1 (See also Plate 9) Rash on patient's legs.

Questions

1. What is the differential diagnosis of choreiform movements?
2. What investigations would narrow the differential and elucidate the diagnosis?
3. What is the most likely diagnosis?
4. What is the significance of the rash (Fig. 13.1), the chorea, and the thrombo-cytopenia?
5. How would you treat her at this stage? How may this change in the future?

Answers

1. What is the differential diagnosis of choreiform movements?

Choreiform movements are likely to result from basal ganglia pathology. The differential diagnosis includes the following:

- Infection-related:
  - viral—varicella, HIV, measles, mumps, herpes simplex, Epstein–Barr, cytomegalovirus
  - pertussis, diphtheria
  - Sydenham's chorea
  - bacterial endocarditis
  - Lyme disease
  - mycoplasma.
- Autoimmune/vasculitis:
  - SLE
  - APS
  - BD
  - sarcoid.
- Vascular:
  - arteriovenous malformation
  - basal ganglia infarction or haemorrhage.
- Endocrine:
  - hyperthyroidism
  - hypoparathyroidism, pseudo-hypoparathyroidism.
- Metabolic:
  - hypocalcaemia
  - hypoglycaemia
  - renal failure
  - hypomagnesaemia
  - hypo- or hypernatraemia.
- Neoplastic:
  - primary and metastatic brain tumour
  - primary CNS lymphoma
  - paraneoplastic syndrome.
- Drug-related:
  - anticholinergics
  - anticonvulsants

- antidopaminergics
- antihistamines
- CNS stimulants
- dopamine agonists
- lithium.
- Epilepsy
- Inherited conditions e.g. Wilson's disease.

2. What investigations would narrow the differential and elucidate the diagnosis?

- Infection screen including viral studies, blood cultures, throat swab, antistrep-tolysin-O titre (ASOT), and an echocardiogram.
- Autoantibodies to include antinuclear antibody (ANA), extractable nuclear antigen (ENA), complement, immunoglobulins, anticardiolipin antibody(aCL), and anti-β_2-glycoprotein-I antibody
- Clotting studies, lupus anticoagulant (LA)
- Urine dipstick for protein and blood, microscopy for casts
- MRI brain
- Lumbar puncture

Investigations showed the following:

- Hb 10.6 g/dL; MCV 79 fL; platelets 58×10^9/L; WCC 6.8×10^9/L with lymphocytes 2.2×10^9/L; ESR 4 mm/h
- Prolonged clotting: PT 15.4 s; activated partial thromboplastin time (APTT) 66.7 s
- Positive LA; aCL 27 IU/ml
- Positive ANA and negative ENA; C3 88 mg/dL (65–190); C4 11.8 mg/dL (14–40)
- CRP <8 mg/L
- Renal and liver function were normal
- Viral studies and ASOT were negative
- Echocardiogram showed mild mitral regurgitation with minor thickening of atrium mitral leaflet and absence of left ventricular or left atrial enlargement.
- MRI excluded focal lesions in the basal ganglia.

3. What is the most likely diagnosis? What is the significance of the rash (Figure 13.1), the chorea, and the thrombocytopenia?

This patient had positive LA and antiphospholipid, with clinical manifestations of anti-phospholipid syndrome (APS), but did not satisfy the classification criteria for the syndrome since she did not have a history of arterial or venous thrombosis.

APS is a non-inflammatory autoimmune disease characterized by recurrent arterial and venous thrombosis and pregnancy-related complications for mother and

Table 13.1 Sapporo Classification Criteria for the antiphospholipid syndrome

Clinical criteria

1. Vascular thrombosis—arterial, venous, or small vessel thrombosis in any tissue or organ
2. Pregnancy morbidity, when other causes have been excluded:

   one or more unexplained deaths at or beyond the 10th week gestation

   one or more premature births before the 34th week of gestation due to eclampsia, severe pre-eclampsia, or placental insufficiency

   three or more consecutive spontaneous abortions before the 10th week of gestation

Laboratory criteria—present on two or more occasions at least 12 weeks apart, in titre >99th percentile

1. Lupus anticoagulant (LA) present in plasma
2. Anticardiolipin (aCL) antibody of IgG and/or IgM isotype in serum or plasma
3. Anti-β_2-glycoprotein-I antibody of IgG and/or IgM isotype in serum or plasma

fetus, and the presence of antiphospholipid antibodies. It can occur as primary APS but is also associated with other autoimmune conditions, most commonly SLE. It occurs mainly in young women, with a male-to-female ratio of 1:3.5 for primary disease and 1:7 in patients with SLE.

The Sapporo criteria (Table 13.1) classify APS as being present if at least one clinical and one laboratory criterion are met. A diagnosis requires the presence of laboratory criteria on two separate occasions 12 weeks apart because only persistent abnormalities are clinically relevant. Although the criteria are not validated in children, they are used for diagnosis as in adults. An international registry of paediatric APS patients has demonstrated 50% as having an underlying autoimmune disease.

Her rash (Fig. 13.1) was livedo reticularis, which is more prevalent among APS patients with SLE and in females.

Non-criteria clinical manifestations of APS include (percentages taken from the Euro-Phospholipid Project):

- livedo reticularis (24%)
- thrombocytopenia (30%)
- neurological manifestations (epilepsy 10%, chorea 1.3%)
- heart valve disease (14%)
- nephropathy (3%).

Livedo reticularis is a violaceous reticular or mottled pattern of the skin on the trunk, arms, or legs. In APS, it occurs predominantly in females with SLE. Histology shows partial or complete occlusion of small to medium-sized arteries and arterioles with no perivascular inflammatory infiltrate and negative direct immunofluorescence examination. The lesions can lead to ischaemia and tissue infarction, termed livedo vasculitis, which manifest as purpura, nodules, and painful ulcers.

Thrombocytopenia is a well-recognized feature of APS, being present in a third of patients. Patients with APS associated with SLE more frequently exhibit thrombocytopenia and leucopenia. Platelet levels are seldom low enough to be associated with haemorrhage and usually function well. Evan's syndrome occurs in some patients with APS and thrombocytopenia who also develop haemolytic anaemia with a positive direct Coombs' test.

The most common neurological manifestations of APS, such as stroke, transient ischaemic attack, and cerebral venous sinus thrombosis are caused by thrombosis. In some cases this may be caused by emboli from cardiac valve vegetations. Not all neurological manifestations are clearly linked to thrombosis; these include chorea, transverse myelopathy, Guillain–Barré syndrome, psychosis, and migraine. Antiphospholipid antibodies may also have specific non-thrombogenic effects on peripheral and central nervous system tissues; for example, anti-β_2-glycoprotein-I has been shown to bind to neuronal and astrocyte membranes.

Heart valve lesions in the form of sessile vegetations or valve thickenings occur in 30–50% patients with APS. This can cause stenosis or regurgitation. Valvular thickening tends to be diffuse, in contrast with the localized thickening of rheumatic heart disease. Cardiac valvular disease contributes to the risk of stroke.

Antiphospholipid antibodies are associated with a renal small artery vasculopathy and chronic renal ischaemia.

SLE should also be considered as a diagnosis in this case. It is important to determine whether an autoimmune disorder is present, as complications such as thrombosis or pregnancy losses may be caused by factors other than those related to APS. Clinical and laboratory features of APS are the same in both APS and APS associated with SLE. The presence of antiphospholipid is frequent in paediatric SLE (55%) and represents a risk factor for thrombosis and poor prognosis overall. This patient had a positive ANA, aCL, LA, and thrombocytopenia, in keeping with SLE, but she did not completely satisfy the criteria for the disease. Later, she developed a malar rash, Raynaud's triad, and a raised anti-double-stranded DNA, supporting a diagnosis of SLE.

4. How would you treat her at this stage? How may this change in the future?

Coexisting risk factors for thrombosis should be identified in every case and used to assess risk. These include increased age (>55 years in men and >65 years in women), inherited thrombophilias, nephrotic syndrome, malignancy, immobilization, surgery, and other cardiovascular risk factors (hypertension, diabetes mellitus, elevated LDL or low HDL cholesterol, smoking, family history of premature cardiovascular disease, body mass index (BMI) >30 kg/m^2, microalbuminuria, reduced estimated GFR of <60mL/min).

VTE with APS should be treated with unfractionated or low molecular weight heparin for at least 5 days overlapped with warfarin adjusted to a target international normalized ratio (INR) of 2–3. The expert consensus view is to anticoagulate these patients indefinitely because of the high rate of recurrence after discontinuation of warfarin.

Arterial thromboembolism most commonly involves the cerebral circulation in the form of stroke or transient ischaemia. The Antiphospholipid Antibodies and

Stroke Study demonstrated no difference in the risk of thrombotic events in patients treated with warfarin and aspirin, and no difference in the risk of bleeding for patients with or without LA or aCL. Patients with a single event may be treated with aspirin 325 mg daily or moderate-intensity warfarin (INR 1.4–2.8).

Women with APS and a history of two or more early pregnancy losses or one or more late pregnancy loss with no prior history of thrombosis should have combination aspirin and heparin during pregnancy. Aspirin should be started with attempted conception and heparin when a viable intra-uterine pregnancy is documented and continued until late in the third trimester.

This case was initially treated with aspirin 75 mg and carbamazepine, and her chorea slowly resolved. Following a further event and MRI evidence of a high signal lesion, likely to be due to ischaemia, indefinite anticoagulation with warfarin was commenced with a target INR of 2.0–3.0. Her SLE was treated with azathioprine and hydroxychloroquine, with resolution of her thrombocytopenia and anaemia.

She will need advice to reduce her risks of thromboembolic disease including discussion of contraception, smoking, and weight gain. She should be aware of the risks of warfarin including interaction with other drugs such as alcohol. She should avoid the oestrogen-containing combined oral contraceptive pill, but it should be safe for her to use the progesterone-only pill. She will need counselling about the increased risk of thrombosis in pregnancy. In view of her mitral valve lesions, she was advised to have prophylaxis for endocarditis.

Further reading

APASS Writing Committee (2004). Antiphospholipid antibodies and subsequent thrombo-occlusive events in patients with ischaemic stroke. *JAMA*; **291**: 576–84.

Buller HR, Agnelli G, Hull RD, Hyers TM, Prins MH, Raskob GE (2004). Antithrombotic therapy for venous thromboembolic disease: the Seventh ACCP Conference on Antithrombotic and Thrombolytic Therapy. *Chest*; **126** (3 Suppl): 401S–28S.

Cervera R, Boffa M-C, Khamashta MA, Hughes GRV (2009). The Euro-Phospholipid Project: epidemiology of the antiphospholipid syndrome in Europe. *Lupus*; **18**: 889–93.

Cohen D, Berger SP, Steup-Beekman GM, Bloemenkamp KWM, Bajema IM (2010). Diagnosis and management of the antiphospholipid syndrome. *BMJ*; **340** c2541.

Lim W, Crowther MA, Eikelboom JW (2006). Management of antiphospholipid antibody syndrome: a systematic review. *JAMA*; **295**: 1050–7.

Miyakis S, Lockshin MD, Atsumi T, *et al.* (2006). International consensus statement on an update of the classification criteria for definite antiphospholipid syndrome (APS). *J Thromb Haemost*; **4**: 295–306.

Ticani A, Branch W, Levy RA, *et al.* (2003). Treatment of pregnant patients with antiphospholipid syndrome. *Lupus*; **12**: 524–9.

Case 14

A 30-year-old female sustained a right tibial fracture whilst walking. She had a history of JIA diagnosed at the age of 4 years which had been difficult to control. She had required prolonged courses of oral corticosteroids and was subsequently treated with methotrexate, alendronate, and calcium and vitamin D supplementation. She was thin, with a BMI of 17 kg/m², and had active synovitis of her wrists. Her menstruation was erratic but she did not have amenorrhea. Her fracture failed to unite, and she required multiple surgical procedures including a bone graft following an infected non-union.

Investigations showed the following:

♦ Hb 11.0 g/dL; WCC 4.73 × 10⁹/L; platelets 234 × 10⁹/L

♦ CRP 13 mg/L; creatinine 43 umol/L; ALP 237 IU/L; ALT 15 IU/L

♦ Calcium 2.3 mmol/L; phosphate 1.23 mmol/L; albumin 44 g/L; parathyroid hormone 2.6 pmol/L (1.3–7.6)

♦ Hormone and thyroid function tests (TFTs) were normal

♦ DEXA scan results:
  • spine—T score –1.7; Z score –1.5
  • hip—T score –1.9; Z score –1.9.

Questions

1. What factors may have contributed to her fracture?
2. How should she be investigated?
3. What should be considered in planning her treatment?

Answers

1. What factors may have contributed to her fracture?

The most likely cause of her low-impact fracture is osteoporosis since she has a low BMD and normal bone markers. Her DEXA scan results show her bone density to be in the osteopenic range but other contributory risk factors are:

- JIA
- prolonged courses of corticosteroids
- low BMI and poor nutritional intake.

Low BMD and fragility fractures are recognized complications of JIA which may persist into adulthood, causing an increased fracture risk compared with the healthy population. It is due to a combination of factors including prolonged inflammation, growth impairment, and reduced physical activity as well as treatment with corticosteroids.

Oral glucocorticoid use is associated with a significant increase in fracture risk which rises rapidly after the onset of treatment and declines after stopping. The increase in fracture risk is over and above the effect of low BMD. Mechanisms include osteoblast dysfunction, osteocyte apoptosis, and disturbed calcium home-ostasis. This patient had stopped her treatment with steroids more than a year prior to fracture, but it is not possible to quantify the effect of years of steroid treatment during growth periods.

Other causes of low-impact fracture include osteomalacia and, in an older patient, malignancies including myeloma. Methotrexate-related osteopathy may be considered as a rare and idiosyncratic triad of severe distal tibial pain, oste-oporosis, and multiple compression fractures.

2. How should she be investigated?

The main principles in investigating and managing a case of osteoporosis are:

- exclusion of diseases mimicking osteoporosis
- identification of the causes and contributory factors
- assessment of the risk of subsequent fracture
- selection of treatment.

Investigations should be selected to confirm the diagnosis of osteoporosis and identify any contributory factors to her low bone density. This is important in planning her treatment to promote bone healing and prevent further fractures. Investigations may include a serum hormone profile (prolactin, oestradiol, proges-terone, follicle-stimulating hormone (FSH), luteinizing hormone (LH), thyroid-stimulating hormone (TSH)) and a 24-hour cortisol–dexamethasone suppression test. In men with osteoporosis, serum testosterone and sex-hormone-binding globulin (SHBG) should be measured. Coeliac disease should be excluded with endomysial or tissue transglutaminase antibodies. Her urinary calcium excretion should be measured and markers of bone turnover, such as P1NP, may be used in assessing her response to treatment. Further imaging, including X-ray or MRI of the lumbar or thoracic spine or isotope bone scans, may be relevant in patients with osteoporosis if further lesions are suspected.

Published guidelines on investigation and treatment of osteoporosis have generally addressed the condition in post-menopausal women and men over 50 years of age. The fracture risk assessment tool (FRAX™) uses clinical risk factors to provide a 10-year probability of a major osteoporotic fracture (spine, hip, forearm, or humerus). It gives guidance on the need for further assessment by DEXA scan and on treatment. The more recently published QFractureScores extend risk assessments to the younger population. There are few data on managing the condition in young women, where the adaptation of available guidelines also needs to consider the long-term effects of treatment on bone health and potential placental transfer of drugs.

Clinical risk factors used for the assessment of fracture probability include age, gender, BMI, previous fragility fracture or parental history of hip fracture, current glucocorticoid treatment, smoking, alcohol intake, and secondary causes of osteoporosis. These include inflammatory arthritis (e.g. rheumatoid arthritis and in this case uncontrolled JIA), untreated hypogonadism, prolonged immobility, organ transplantation, type 1 diabetes, hyperthyroidism, gastrointestinal or chronic liver disease, and chronic obstructive pulmonary disease.

3. What should be considered in planning her treatment?

Treatment includes advice on lifestyle and pharmacological management. Lifestyle measures to increase bone density should be recommended to all patients with low bone density: weight-bearing exercise, an adequate calcium intake, and avoidance of smoking and excessive alcohol consumption.

The main pharmacological treatments of osteoporosis are the bisphosphonates, strontium ranelate, raloxifene, and parathyroid hormone (PTH) peptides. These should all be prescribed with calcium and vitamin D (see p. 7). Alendronate is the first-line treatment in most cases and is approved for the prevention and treatment of glucocorticoid-induced osteoporosis. There are concerns about the lack of data on the long-term use of bisphosphonates in young women, including the risk of placental transfer.

Bisphosphonates treat osteoporosis by inhibiting osteoclasts and thereby reducing bone resorption. PTH analogues such as teriparatide stimulate the formation and action of osteoblasts responsible for bone formation and promote increases in bone tissue. They are contraindicated for patients at risk of developing osteosarcoma and patients with hyperparthyroidism or hypercalcaemia.

Since this patient was pre-menopausal, all treatment for osteoporosis was unlicensed. She was given advice on improving her nutrition, particularly maintaining a calcium intake of 1000 mg/day, a vitamin D intake of 800 IU/day, and a protein intake of 1 g/kg body weight. She was advised to increase her BMI to >19 kg/m². Measures were taken to improve control of her inflammatory disease. She had previously taken alendronate for 2 years prior to her fracture. Following non-union of her fracture she was treated with teriparatide.

Further reading

Hippisley-Cox J, Coupland C (2009). Predicting risk of osteoporotic fracture in men and women in England and Wales: prospective derivation and validation of QFractureScores. *BMJ*; **339**: b4229 doi: 10.1136/bmj.b4229.

Kanis JA, Johnell O, Odan A, Johannson H, McCloskey E (2008). FRAX and the assessment of fracture probability in men and women from the UK. *Osteoporos Int*; **19**: 385–97.

National Osteoporosis Guideline Group (2008). *Guideline for the Diagnosis and Management of Osteoporosis in Postmenopausal Women and Men from the Age of 50 Years in the UK*. Available online at: www.shef.ac.uk/NOGG.

Royal College of Physicians, Bone and Tooth Society of Great Britain, National Osteoporosis Society (2002). *Glucocorticoid-induced Osteoporosis: Guidelines for Prevention and Treatment*. London: Royal College of Physicians.

Thornton J, Ashcroft D, O'Neill T, *et al.* (2008). A systematic review of the effectiveness of strategies for reducing fracture risk in children with juvenile idiopathic arthritis with additional data on long-term risk of fracture and cost of disease management. *Health Technol Assess*; **12**: 1–208.

Case 15

A one-year-old child presented to the paediatric on-call team with a 5-week history of high spiking temperatures, weight loss, marked irritability, a widespread rash, and a limp. On examination, his heart rate was 140 beats/min and his temperature was 38.2°C. Chest examination was otherwise normal. He had hepatomegaly and symmetrical bilateral wrist swelling.

Investigations showed the following:

◆ Hb 9 g/dL; WCC 39.27 × 10⁹/L; platelets 806 × 10⁹/L; ESR 46 mm/h

◆ CRP 160 mg/L; ferritin 1650 μg/L; ALT 31 U/L; ALP 390 U/L; triglycerides 0.9 mmol/L

A CT scan of the chest is shown in Fig. 15.1.

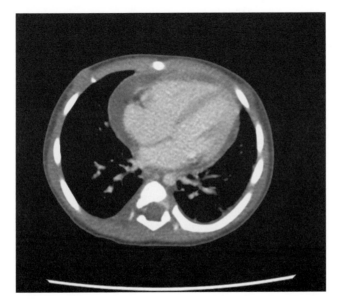

Fig. 15.1 CT scan of chest.

He was admitted to hospital and started treatment. Ten days later he remained extremely unwell and irritable. His temperature was now persistently raised above 39°C. Investigations now showed the following:

- Hb 7.9 g/dL; WCC 67.37 × 10⁹/L; platelets 230 × 10⁹/L; ESR 9.
- CRP 120 mg/L; ALT 1171 U/L; ALP 1226 U/L.
- PT 28.7 s; partial thromboplastin time (PTT) 41.7 s.

Questions

1. Give some causes of pyrexia in a child? What is the most likely diagnosis in this child at presentation?

2. What does the CT scan show?

3. What is the management of the initial condition?

4. What is the likely cause of his deterioration and what is the management of this complication?

Answers

1. Give some causes of pyrexia in a child? What is the most likely diagnosis in this child at presentation?

Causes of pyrexia in a child include:

◆ Infection

◆ Malignancy such as acute lymphoblastic leukaemia

◆ IBD,

◆ Systemic-onset juvenile idiopathic arthritis (SOJIA),

◆ Connective tissue disease such as SLE

◆ Vasculitis such as Kawasaki disease,

◆ Castleman's disease (giant lymph node hyperplasia)

◆ Periodic fever such as FMF.

Fever is a common sign of illness in children and when prolonged beyond 2 weeks is termed pyrexia of unknown origin (PUO). Investigation includes a full infection screen, echocardiography, bone marrow examination, serum lactate dehydrogenase (LDH), urate, and urinalysis for catecholamines.

Recurrent bouts of fever may be associated with a number of rheumatological disorders, including BD and SLE, as well as the hereditary periodic fever syndromes. Leukaemia may present with musculoskeletal pain and arthritis; typically there is diffuse pain and tenderness in the long bones, migratory joint pain and swelling, and systemic features including low-grade fever and weight loss. The full blood count may be normal or demonstrate abnormal white cell or platelet counts. There may be increased inflammatory markers and LDH and urate levels. A neuroblastoma may present with bone metastases and fever, and high urinary vanillylmandelic acid and homovanillic acid support the diagnosis. Recurrent fever may occur in IBD, associated with diarrhoea, anaemia, and growth delay. Kawasaki disease is one of the most common vasculitides of childhood and is an important differential. It generally presents under the age of 5 years with fever, bilateral conjunctival injection, oropharyngeal mucous membrane changes (fissured lips and strawberry tongue), a polymorphous rash, cervical lymphadenopathy, and erythema and oedema of the hands and feet, resulting in periungual desquamation. Castleman's disease is rare in children and presents with diffuse lymphadenopathy and systemic symptoms. The hereditary periodic fever syndromes are autoinflammatory diseases affecting the innate immune system. Episodes of pyrexia generally last days and may be associated with rash, abdominal pain, headache, and joint symptoms. There may be a family history and immunology is negative.

This child presented with evidence of systemic inflammation, rash, and a spiking temperature lasting for weeks. The development of arthritis supported the diagnosis of SOJIA. It is included in the classification of JIA and is defined as arthritis in one or more joints preceded by at least 2 weeks by a quotidian fever and accompanied by a non-fixed evanescent erythematous macular rash, generalized lymphadenopathy, hepatomegaly or splenomegaly, and serositis. It is characterized by marked extra-articular features. The quotidian fever associated with SOJIA differs from that due to sepsis by a return to normal at least once during each 24 hours and it must be present for 2 weeks. It characteristically occurs in association with the development of a discrete, pink, non-pruritic macular rash occurring in crops over the trunk and limbs which may exhibit Koebner's phenomenon. Laboratory features include a hypochromic normocytic anaemia, leucocytosis, and thrombocytosis. The ESR, CRP, and ferritin levels are usually high.

The aetiology of SOJIA is unclear but it resembles the autoinflammatory syndromes and appears to be related to an abnormal genetic coding for proinflammatory proteins. High serum levels of tumour necrosis factor (TNF) and interleukins 6 and 1 (IL-6 and IL-1) have been demonstrated in the sera of patients with the condition.

2. What does the CT scan show?

The CT scan (Fig. 15.1) shows a small pericardial effusion. Pericardial effusions occur in 3–9% of SOJIA cases and are usually asymptomatic, although some children have dyspnoea or precordial pain. It may be evident on examination by diminished heart sounds, tachycardia, cardiomegaly, and a pericardial friction rub at the left lower sternal border.

3. What is the management of the initial condition?

Depending on severity, the management of SOJIA may include the following:

- NSAIDS (e.g. ibuprofen 10 mg/kg three times daily).
- high-dose oral steroids (prednisolone 2 mg/kg/day).
- intravenous methylprednisolone 10–30 mg/kg/day for 1–3 days, followed by oral prednisolone.
- methotrexate 15–20 mg/m^2 weekly for long-term control of articular disease, although it may be less effective in controlling systemic symptoms.

Biological agents against IL-6 and IL-1 have been used with some success when the systemic features are marked.

4. What is the likely cause of his deterioration and what is the management of this complication?

The deterioration in his condition with the development of persistent fever raised concerns that he was developing macrophage activation syndrome (MAS). This is a severe and potentially life-threatening syndrome characterized by fever, pancytopenia, hepatosplenomegaly, lymphadenopathy, elevated liver transaminases, intravascular coagulation, and CNS dysfunction. Triglycerides and ferritin are raised, PT and PTT are prolonged, and ESR is paradoxically low in association with hypofibrinoginaemia. MAS is associated with SOJIA, SLE, and polyarticular JIA. It may be triggered by infection with members of the herpesvirus family, including EBV, or drugs including gold, NSAIDs, hydroxychloroquine, and D-penicillamine.

MAS is a form of secondary haemophagocytic lymphohistiocytosis, but differs from the classical form of this disease in a number of ways, presenting with a relative rather than absolute decrease in white cell count, platelets, or fibrinogen. Bone marrow aspirate may not demonstrate haemophagocytosis early in the disease. In this case, the WCC count remained high but MAS was indicated by the low ESR, raised triglycerides, and falling haemoglobin and platelets.

The treatment of MAS is with:

◆ high-dose parenteral corticosteroids

◆ ciclosporin 4 mg/kg/day.

Biological agents such as etanercept, anakinra, and tocilizumab have also been used with variable results.

This patient had an incomplete response to intravenous corticosteroids and was treated with anakinra. He made a good recovery and was managed in the longer term with subcutaneous weekly injections of methotrexate 20 mg/m^2.

Further reading

Hull RG on behalf of the British Paediatric Rheumatology Group (2001). Guidelines for management of childhood arthritis. *Rheumatology*; **40**: 1309–12.

Petty RE, Southwood TR, Manners P, *et al.* (2004). International League of Associations for Rheumatology classification of juvenile idiopathic arthritis: second revision, Edmonton, 2001. *J Rheumatol*; **31**: 390–2.

Ravelli A (2002). Macrophage activation syndrome. *Curr Opin Rheumatol*; **14**: 548–52.

Ravelli A, Magni-Manzoni S, Pistorio A, *et al.* (2005). Preliminary diagnostic guidelines for macrophage activation syndrome complicating systemic juvenile idiopathic arthritis. *J Paediatr*; **146**: 598–604.

Woo P (2006). Systemic juvenile idiopathic arthritis: diagnosis, management, and outcome. *Nature Clinical Practice*; **2**, 28–34.

Case 16

A 67-year-old man with a 26-year history of AS presented to the rheumatology clinic with increased pain in his back. Four months previously he had been admitted under the general medical team after collapsing at home. A diagnosis of pulmonary embolism was made and confirmed on a computed tomography pulmonary angiogram (CTPA). The patient was discharged home on wafarin, but continued to have severe pain in his back. The pain was not alleviated by exercise, prevented sleep, and was very debilitating.

There was no history of weight loss or systemic features of infection, and the patient had no prior treatment with immunosuppressive therapy. His analgesia included diclofenac 50 mg three times daily and morphine sulphate tablets 10 mg twice daily, with breakthough Oramorph as required.

Examination revealed a moderate kyphosis. He was tender to palpation over T12–L3 with restricted hip movement and no evidence of peripheral synovitis. The patient was afebrile and systems examination was unremarkable, including intact neurology. His Bath Ankylosing Spondylitis Disease Activity Index (BASDAI) score was 6/10 and his spinal pain Visual Analogue Score (VAS) was 9/10 cm.

Investigations showed the following:

- Hb 13.5 g/dL; WCC 7.7 × 10^9/L; platelets 192 × 10^9/L; creatinine 110 µmol/L
- CRP 8 mg/L, ESR 4 mm/h.

MRI of the spine is shown in Fig. 16.1.

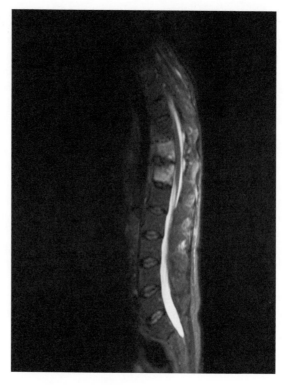

Fig. 16.1 T$_2$-weighted sagittal MRI of spine.

Questions

1. What is your differential diagnosis of the back pain?
2. What does the MR scan show?
3. How would you manage this patient?
4. Would you consider this patient for biological therapy?
5. What are the current NICE guidelines for the treatment of AS with biological therapy?

Answers

1. What is your differential diagnosis of the back pain?

The patient has a raised BASDAI and spinal VAS which could indicate a flare in his inflammatory back pain. However, the pain is more mechanical in nature, i.e. it does not settle with exercise and there is point tenderness over the spine. A recent pulmonary embolism may suggest an undiagnosed malignancy with secondary metastases in the spine. Other differentials include an acute discitis or osteomyelitis, although the normal CRP and lack of fever would argue against this.

Finally, the patient sustained a fall when he collapsed at home, so he should be investigated for a fracture.

2. What does the MR scan show?

The MRI of the spine demonstrates high signal in the vertebral bodies of T11 and T12 extending into the posterior elements, with collapse of the superior endplate of T12 and the inferior endplate of T11. The findings would be in keeping with a traumatic Andersson lesion, or pseudo-arthrosis, involving the posterior elements. The lack of high signal in the disc space itself makes infection unlikely. There is extrusion of the disc material anteriorly and the anterior longitudinal ligament is displaced. There is no evidence of spinal canal stenosis and the cord signal is normal. The diagnosis of AS is confirmed by the partial fusion of the lumbar and thoracic vertebrae. Standard CT allows better evaluation of fractures and destructive vertebral lesions than MRI of the spine and was subsequently performed in this case (Fig. 16.2). This confirmed AS with a T11/12 Andersson lesion as the cause of the sudden-onset back pain in this patient.

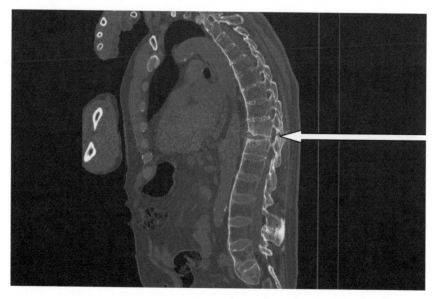

Fig. 16.2 Sagittal CT image of spine showing Andersson lesion (arrow).

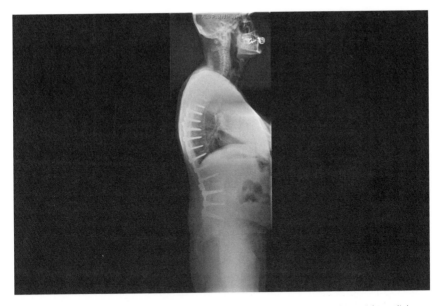

Fig. 16.3 X-ray of whole spine showing extensive spinal instrumentation with pedicle screws from the upper thoracic to the lower lumbar region. The rods bridge the pseudo-arthrosis in the upper lumbar spine.

3. How would you manage this patient?

This patient's spine is unstable with an increased risk of spinal cord compression if left untreated. Surgical fixation is the treatment of choice, and the outcome is shown in Fig. 16.3. The possible complications of spinal surgery include damage to the spinal cord or spinal nerves in addition to general risks including anaesthetic complications, bleeding, thrombosis, dural tear, infection, and persistent pain.

4. Would you consider this patient for biological therapy?

Although this patient has raised BASDAI and spinal VAS scores, these can be attributed to the pseudo-arthrosis rather than reflecting inflammatory disease activity. This patient would be unlikely to benefit from biological therapy and treatment should focus on surgical correction, appropriate analgesia, and physiotherapy postoperatively.

5. What are the current NICE guidelines for the treatment of AS with biological therapy?

NICE guidance recommends the use of the TNF inhibitors adalimumab and etanercept as treatment options in adults with severe active AS. There are three elements that should be satisfied before a patient is eligible for anti-TNF therapy.

First, the Modified New York Criteria for the diagnosis of AS must be satisfied, including the radiological criterion and at least one clinical criterion.

◆ Clinical criteria:
  • low back pain present for >3 months, improved by exercise but not relieved by rest
  • limitation of lumbar spine motion in sagittal and frontal planes
  • limitation of chest expansion relative to normal values for age and sex.
◆ Radiological criterion:
  • sacroiliitis on radiographs.

Further, there must be evidence of sustained active spinal disease, which is confirmed by:

◆ score of ≥4 units on BASDAI

◆ score of ≥ 4 cm on the 0–10 cm spinal pain VAS.

These scores must be measured twice, at least 12 weeks apart, on stable treatment.

Lastly, patients should have failed treatment with at least two different conventional NSAIDs taken at maximum tolerated or recommended dosages for 4 weeks respectively.

Exclusion criteria for the use of anti-TNF agents include patients with active significant infection, a septic arthritis of a native joint within the last 12 months, prosthetic joint infection within the last 12 months or indefinitely if the prosthesis if not removed, New York Heart Association (NYHA) grade 3 or 4 congestive cardiac failure (CCF), history of demyelinating disease, women who are pregnant or breastfeeding, and malignancy.

Patients who are started on anti-TNF therapy must be assessed 12 weeks after starting treatment. An adequate response is defined as a 50% reduction or a reduction by ≥2 units in BASDAI, and a reduction in the spinal pain VAS by ≥2 cm. Patients who reach this response are eligible to continue treatment with anti-TNF therapy.

If patients are intolerant to a specific anti-TNF therapy, for example due to injection site reactions, then they are eligible to switch to another, but under NICE they cannot switch because of lack of efficacy alone.

At present, the published NICE guidance does not recommend the use of infliximab in the treatment of AS, although if patients are already receiving the treatment they have the option to continue. This is in contrast to the British Society for Rheumatology (BSR) guidelines (2006) which recommend the use of infliximab as an option for treating patients with AS.

Further reading

Keat A, Barkham N, Bhalla A, *et al.* on behalf of the BSR Standards, Guidelines, and Audit Working Group (2005). BSR guideline for prescribing TNF-α blockers in adults with ankylosing spondylitis. Report of a working party of the British Society for Rheumatology. *Rheumatology*; **44**: 939–47.

Kim KT, Lee SH, Suk KS, Lee JH, Im YJ (2007). Spinal pseudoarthrosis in advanced ankylosing spondylitis with sagittal plane deformity. *Spine*; **32**: 1641–7.

NICE (2008). Adalimumab, etanercept and infliximab for ankylosing spondylitis. *NICE Technology Appraisal Guidance 143*. Available from: http://guidance.nice.org.uk/TA143.

Case 17

A 24-year-old male competitive 800 m runner presented with a 6-week history of left posterior heel pain and swelling. The pain had started insidiously with no specific injury. The pain was now constant at mild to moderate intensity but significantly worse during and for a few hours after running. He had changed coaches 2 months previously and had modified his training programme to include more speed work.

He had tried ice massage to his heel and oral NSAIDs with limited benefit.

His past medical history included a motor vehicle accident 2 years previously. This had resulted in chronic lower back pain and morning stiffness.

Examination revealed over-pronation of his hindfoot during walking and running. There was mild swelling and moderate tenderness over the insertion of the left Achilles tendon into the calcaneus. Lower back movement was restricted in all planes. A modified Schöber's test gave a result of +3 cm. There was no discomfort on stressing the sacroiliac joints. A few red scaly patches were noted on the back of his scalp.

Investigations showed the following:

- CRP 7 mg/L
- Ultrasound of left Achilles tendon: irregular fusiform swelling of the distal portion of the tendon at the inserted into the calcaneus with mild hypoechoic echotexture and loss of fibrillar pattern associated small bony heel spur
- His HLA B27 status was negative.

Questions

1. What is the differential diagnosis?
2. What further information might be helpful in making a diagnosis?
3. Are there any other investigations you would like to perform? How would these help?
4. How would you manage this patient?

Answers

1. What is the differential diagnosis?

He has an insertional Achilles tendinopathy. The two most likely differential diagnoses are:

- mechanical overuse tendinopathy
- enthesitis related to a spondyloarthropathy (e.g. psoriatic arthropathy).

Mechanical overuse tendinopathy is a degenerative condition thought to be the result of repetitive strain which causes chronic micro-tears to the tendon. Tendons continuously slowly remodel to adapt to the loads placed upon them. If they are unable to adapt, tendinopathy can develop. The histological features are hypertrophy of fibroblasts, abundant disorganized collagen, and vascular hyperplasia. This does not involve inflammatory cells and therefore the term tendonitis is misleading. The mechanism of the pain is poorly understood.

Running is one of the most common causes of a mechanical overuse tendinopathy of the Achilles tendon. Excessive motion of the hindfoot due to lateral heel strike and over-pronation can cause a whipping action of the Achilles tendon and predispose it to injury. Recent changes to running technique, increased training intensity, and new or worn footwear can be precipitating factors. The most common area for Achilles tendinopathy to develop in an athlete is in the mid-portion (2–6 cm proximal to the tuber calcanei). Only about 20% of mechanical Achilles tendinopathies are insertional. Insertional tendinopathies are often associated with retro-calcaneal bursitis and/or Haglund's deformity (bony enlargement of the back of the calcaneus). Tendinopathy is also common in the non-athletic population, particularly in people who are overweight and have biomechanical lower-limb problems.

In this patient an enthesitis related to an inflammatory spondyloarthropathy needs to be considered in view of his chronic low back pain and morning stiffness. Less than 30% of patients with psoriatic arthritis are positive for HLA B27.

2. What further information might be helpful in making a diagnosis?

It is important to ascertain whether he had back symptoms prior to his motor vehicle accident. It is also pertinent to ask about other symptoms which might suggest spondyloarthritis such as peripheral arthritis, dactylitis, psoriasis, palmar plantar pustulosis, balanitis, nail changes, other recurrent tendon problems, iritis, or inflammatory bowel symptoms. Enquiries should be made about a family history of psoriasis and inflammatory arthritis.

3. Are there any other investigations you would like to perform? How would these help?

Consider imaging the sacroiliac joints and lumbar/thoracic spine with an MRI scan. Features of sacroiliitis (bone oedema, synovitis, erosion, and sclerosis) may be visible on MRI if the underlying aetiology is psoriatic arthritis or ankylosing spondylitis. Romanus lesions at the corners of the vertebral body may be present in the lumbar or thoracic spine. These appear as bright signal on STIR MRI sequences and indicate enthesitis of the spinal ligament insertion to the vertebral body. Ultrasound of the tendon is useful to monitor improvement over time, but is unlikely to differentiate between insertional mechanical overuse tendinopathy and enthesitis from a spondyloarthropathy. Thickening of the tendon insertion, calcific deposits, periosteal changes, and vascularization (seen by Doppler ultrasound) can be found in both settings.

4. How would you manage this patient?

Treatment will be guided by whether or not the insertional tendinopathy is thought to be mechanical or inflammatory in aetiology:

Mechanical overuse

i) Relative rest from activities causing the problem (in this case time off from running).

ii) Eccentric calf raises. This is a well-established therapy for mid-portion Achilles tendinopathy but has not been very successful in insertional tendinopathies. In the original studies with eccentric training the patient did the exercise on a step and the heel went lower than the rest of the foot, causing dorsiflexion at the ankle. It is now thought that dorsiflexion causes impingement between tendon, bursa, and bone at the insertion, resulting in a compressive force, and hence is the reason for treatment failure in those with insertional tendinonopathy. It has been demonstrated that eccentric calf raises done on flat ground with no dorsiflexion at the ankle improves insertional tendinopathy. Three sets of 15 repetitions with knee straight and three sets of 15 repetitions with knee bent twice a day for 12 weeks are the minimum treatment course.

iii) Correct any biomechanical abnormality. In this patient, correction of overpronation is important, either by using support shoes or by referral for orthotics to have medial arch supports made to fit his running shoes.

iv) A variety of 'novel' treatments are currently used but they have little or no evidence base at present. Sclerotherapy has been used to reduce the 'neovascularization' which is thought to contribute to the pain. Dry needling, autologous blood, and platelet-rich plasma (PRP) injections are also in use. The rationale is that the trauma and blood/PRP provides the growth factors necessary for tendon repair. Extracorporeal shock wave therapy and high-volume tenotomy are also occasionally offered, but the recommendation for these second-line therapies is anecdotal rather than evidence-based.

Inflammatory spondyloarthropathy

i) Education about disease and symptomatic treatment.

ii) Physiotherapy to maintain range of back flexibility.

iii) Anti-inflammatories.

iv) Consider corticosteroid injection into sacroiliac joint if there is sacroiliitis on MRI.

v) Anti-TNF therapy for refractory disease. There is no proven benefit of traditional DMARD therapy in the setting of spinal inflammation or enthesitis. DMARDs can be used if there is an associated peripheral arthritis.

Further reading

Alfredson H (2005). The chronic painful Achilles and patellar tendon: research on basic biology and treatment. *Scand J Med Sci Sports*; **15**: 252–9.

Antoni CE, Kavanaugh A, Kirkham B, *et al.* (2005). Sustained benefits of infliximab therapy for dermatologic and articular manifestations of psoriatic arthritis: results from the Infliximab Multinational Psoriatic Arthritis Controlled Trial (IMPACT). *Arthritis Rheum*; **52**: 1227–36.

Jonsson P, Alfredson H, Sunding K, *et al.* (2008). New regimen for eccentric calf-muscle training in patients with chronic insertional Achilles tendinopathy: results of a pilot study. *Br J Sports Med*; **42**: 746–9.

Case 18

A 26-year-old healthy landscape gardener attended the rheumatology clinic complaining of a year's history of intermittent wrist discomfort, numbness, and pins and needles in his hands. His symptoms had started during a period of heavy gardening.

His past medical history included an injury to his upper spine 6 years previously, which had occurred while using a sledgehammer. These symptoms resolved over a 6-month period. He had a more recent 2-year history of stiffness across his shoulders and upper back.

On examination he had a forward protruding neck at the cervico-thoracic junction, with some restriction of thoracic and scapular mobility. He had a full range of pain-free movement at the wrists and fingers with no swollen or tender joints. Power, tone, reflexes, and sensation in the upper and lower limbs were normal. Tapping the palmar aspect of the wrist over the carpal tunnel to elicit paraesthesia in the distribution of the median nerve (Tinel's test) was negative. However, he reported mild paraesthesia 1.5 minutes into Phalen's test where the wrist is held in a fully flexed position for 2 minutes.

The physiotherapist was able to reproduce his symptoms by stressing the brachial plexus on both sides. The upper thoracic joints were described as hypomobile.

Questions

1. What are the possible causes of the symptoms in his hands?
2. What clinical tests are useful in confirming the diagnosis?
3. How would you manage this patient?

Answers

1. What are the possible causes of the symptoms in his hands?

- Musculoskeletal soft tissue symptoms related to adverse neural dynamics (AND) are the most likely cause of his symptoms in view of his age, neck posture, the intermittent nature of his symptoms, and the absence of other neurological signs.

- Central cervical disc prolapse at C5–6 or C6–7 should be considered in view of his previous history of injury and his symptoms during a period of heavy gardening.

- Bilateral median nerve entrapment is a possible diagnosis in view of his occupation and use of heavy equipment.

- CNS disorders such as demyelination are less likely.

2. What clinical tests are useful in confirming the diagnosis?

'Adverse neural dynamics' may cause symptoms of pain, paraesthesia, or numbness due to the restriction of movement or irritation of the nerve through its course from spine to distal origin. This is seen, for example, with the straight-leg raise and 'slump tests'. Upper-limb neural mobilization tests, usually used by physiotherapists, are used to identify which nerves of the brachial plexus are predominantly affected where upper limb symptoms occur. The patient is examined in the supine position with the hand of the untested side resting on the patient's abdomen. The patient reports any pain, stretching, tingling, or numbness. Figures 18.1–18.3 describe the sequences of testing for median, ulnar, and radial nerves, respectively. A test is deemed positive if the patient's symptoms are at least partially recreated specifically during the mobilization. These symptoms and signs are often present in work-related upper-limb disorders related to repetitive use or overuse activities, such as excessive keyboard work. They can also be seen in patients who suffer whiplash injuries or any musculoskeletal impairment, as in this patient, where soft tissue damage compromises the nerve in its pathway.

The symptoms of AND are common, especially in individuals who use a computer for prolonged periods. It affects men and women equally and can occur at any age.

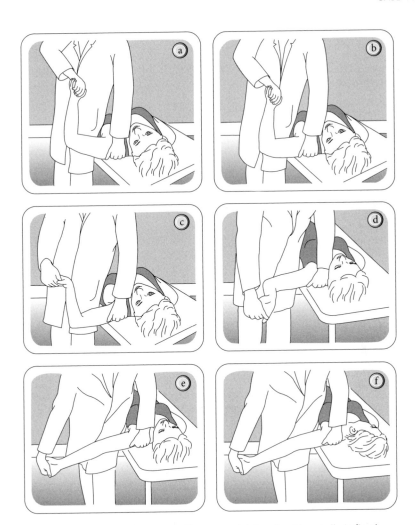

Fig. 18.1 Testing sequence for the median nerve. (a) the shoulder girdle is fixed. (b) the shoulder is abducted. (c) the wrist is extended. (d) the shoulder is externally rotated. (e) the elbow is extended. (f) the head is laterally flexed away from the side being tested.

Adapted from *Mobilisation of the Nervous System*, Butler, DS, p. 149, Copyright Churchill Livingstone (1991).

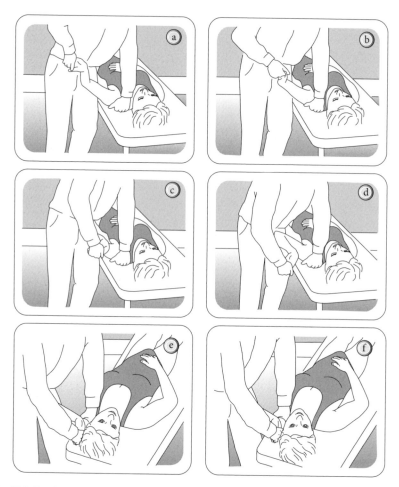

Fig. 18.2 Testing sequence for the ulnar nerve (a) the wrist is extended. (b) the arm is pronated. (c) the elbow is flexed. (d) the shoulder is depressed. (e) the shoulder is externally rotated. (f) the shoulder is abducted.
Adapted from *Mobilisation of the Nervous System*, Butler, DS, pp. 158–9, Copyright Churchill Livingstone (1991).

3. How would you manage this patient?

A patient with AND should be managed with physiotherapy and home posture exercises. This will include correction of posture and muscle balance to improve biomechanics, spinal joint mobilization, soft tissue massage, and exercises and skin taping in order to offload structures and improve local proprioception.

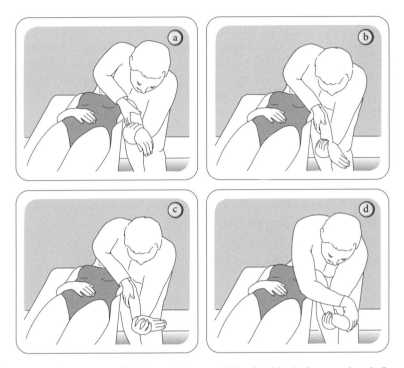

Fig. 18.3 Testing sequence for the radial nerve (a) the shoulder is depressed and elbow extended. (b) the shoulder is internally rotated. (c) the wrist is flexed. (d) the shoulder is abducted.
Adapted from *Mobilisation of the Nervous System*, Butler, DS, p. 155, Copyright Churchill Livingstone (1991).

It is important to address activities that aggravate symptoms, including assessment of the patient's work environment and posture. They may need advice on pacing, splitting repetitive tasks, and reduction of upper-limb use with voice recognition software in the case of keyboard users. He may need to liaise with his employers or managers to ensure that he takes regular breaks at work and may need to change to lighter jobs. If these measures do not resolve his symptoms, he may have to make significant changes to his work.

Further reading

Butler DS (1991). *Mobilisation of the Nervous System*. Melbourne: Churchill Livingstone.

Schmid AB, Brunner F, Luomajoki H, *et al.* (2009). Reliability of clinical tests to evaluate nerve function and mechanosensitivity of the upper limb peripheral nervous system. *BMC Musculoskelet Disord*; **10**: 11 (available from: http://www.ncbi.nlm.nih.gov/pmc/articles/PMC2653029/?tool=pubmed).

Turl SE, George KP (1998). Adverse neural tension: a factor in repetitive hamstring strain? *J Orthop Sports Phys Ther*; **27**: 16–21.

Case 19

A 47-year-old nurse was referred with a 3-month history of dry eyes and mouth and aching upper-arm muscles, and a 3-day history of left-sided facial weakness. For the previous year she had been suffering from fatigue, poor sleep, and non-specific joint pains. Six months previously she had developed a pustular psoriatic rash on her palms and feet, resistant to topical treatments.

She had no antecedent history of infection, arthritis, colitis, or recent foreign travel. She had last visited her family in Nigeria 5 years previously. She was married with two children aged 8 and 10. She had lived in the UK for 5 years.

On examination she had palmar pustular psoriasis, tender deltoid muscles, swollen parotids, and a left lower motor neuron facial nerve palsy. Joint examination was normal with full range of movement and no synovitis. Schirmer's test was positive.

Investigations showed the following:

- Normal FBC
- Normal liver and renal function
- CPK 500 IU/L
- RF and ACCP negative; ANA negative; ENAs negative; ANCA negative; HLA B27 negative; serum ACE normal
- CXR clear.

Questions

1. Suggest a unifying diagnosis.
2. What further information is needed to establish the underlying diagnosis?
3. What treatments are available?
4. What are the implications for her occupation and her family?
5. What musculoskeletal complications may occur in response to treatment?

Answers

1. Suggest a unifying diagnosis

Multisystem inflammatory autoimmune conditions like SLE, primary Sjögren's syndrome, and antisynthetase syndrome are important differential diagnoses. However, her profession and travel from an HIV-endemic area means that HIV/AIDs must be considered. HIV/AIDS would account for the chronic fatigue, late-onset aggressive palmar pustular psoriasis, myositis, and parotid enlargement with facial nerve involvement (diffuse infiltrative lymphocytosis syndrome (DILS)).

Some patients develop symptoms in association with seroconversion. Unexplained arthralgias occur in 5% of HIV-positive patients who also suffer from fibromyalgia-like symptoms. Joint pain may occur in the absence of synovitis. A lower-limb, self-limiting, non-erosive monoarthritis can occur.

Psoriasis, myositis, and DILS can all be initial presentations of HIV infection. Psoriasis may be dramatic and intractable, with poor response to topical treatments.

Myositis is usually subacute and progressive. Skin involvement is rare. EMG studies can be normal or show non-specific, short-duration, polyphasic, motor-unit potentials with abnormal spontaneous activity. Muscle biopsy may show infiltrate of inflammatory cells in necrotic and non-necrotic fibres. Often the lesions are ill-defined. In HIV-positive patients it is important to rule out opportunistic infections such as toxoplasmosis, which can occur during immune compromise and also presents with muscle weakness and raised muscle enzymes.

DILS occurs in 3–4% of HIV-positive patients. Proposed diagnostic criteria for DILS include HIV seropositivity with either bilateral salivary gland enlargement or xerostomia for >6 months. Histology shows lymphocytic infiltration of salivary or lacrimal glands in the absence of granulomatous or neoplastic enlargement. Gadolinium-67 scintigraphy of salivary glands is positive. Inflammatory myopathy and DILS can be associated with infiltrative peripheral neuropathy, lymphocytic hepatitis, and lymphocytic infiltrative pneumonia.

This woman's facial palsy may have been secondary to the parotid gland infiltration.

2. What further information is needed to establish the underlying diagnosis?

A careful history for HIV risk factors includes needle stick injury (UK or abroad), intravenous drug use with needle sharing, and sexual contact with persons at risk of HIV or from HIV-endemic areas.

- The most important test is an HIV test. Combined antigen/antibody tests currently used for screening will detect patients within 4 weeks of exposure. Patients need appropriate counselling and consent before testing.
- 50% of HIV-infected patients in the UK are ignorant of their diagnosis.
- CD4 count is helpful in tracking progress, but it is expensive and should not be used to confirm diagnosis. Assessment for other sexually transmitted diseases and infective hepatitis screening are also needed.

This woman was HIV positive with a CD4 count of 200. Her potential risk factor was her husband who travelled regularly to Africa on business. He refused HIV testing.

3. What treatments are available?

Treatment of HIV is highly specialized and should be conducted under expert supervision. Current standard therapy is highly active antiretroviral therapy (HAART).

Low to moderate-dose steroids may be used to treat glandular swelling and interstitial pneumonia but immunosuppressive therapies, including steroids, need to be used with caution as they may increase viral load and worsen the illness.

Sicca symptoms of dry eyes and mouth are treated symptomatically.

The facial palsy may not respond to treatment and may be permanent.

Psoriasis associated with HIV is often resistant to topical treatments. Methotrexate and ciclosporin may improve skin lesions, but there is increased risk of systemic infection. Hydroxyurea is generally considered a safer alternative. The psoriasis usually settles with HIV treatment.

Explosive reactive arthritis can occur which is difficult to treat with conventional therapy. The association with HLA B27 is less strong, particularly in African populations where the HLA B27 prevalence is low.

4. What are the implications for her occupation and her family?

The patient's immediate family, husband and children, should be tested for HIV. If her children test negative, then their future risk of transmission from her is negligible. Her husband refused HIV testing. Whatever his HIV status, counselling about safe sex and contact tracing is important.

There are implications for future pregnancies, primarily around time of delivery. Strategies taken in the UK and other developed countries have reduced the risk of vertical transmission of HIV from mother to infant to <2%. These strategies involve universal HIV screening of all pregnant women, treating pregnant HIV-positive patients with HAART to make viral load undetectable before delivery, elective Caesarean section; avoidance of breastfeeding, and 6 weeks zidovudine prophylaxis for the infants. In resource-poor countries the advice on breastfeeding is different.

Implications for her employment depend on her workplace. She is safe to work in all environments apart from an 'exposure-prone environment' where she is unable to see her hands and may catch them on a spike of bone or surgical instrument (e.g. assisting some operations in theatre).

She should not work where there is high exposure to tuberculosis. She should have antibody testing for varicella and CMV.

5. What musculoskeletal complications may occur in response to treatment?

Complications of HAART include metabolic abnormalities with lipid abnormalities, insulin resistance, and changes in body fat distribution. Although (low BMD) osteopenia and osteoporosis are frequent in HIV-positive patients, it is still unclear whether this is a direct consequence of the viral infection or of the antiretroviral drugs. Treatment is with bisphosphonates plus calcium and Vitamin D supplementation.

Zidovudine-induced myopathy

Zidovudine (a nucleoside analogue) has been first-line treatment for AIDS since 1987 and is associated with myopathy in 2–18% patients. Patients present with myalgia and muscle weakness and an associated rise in CK. Incidence is minimized by using low-dose zidovudine and monitoring CK levels during treatment. Treatment is to withdraw zidovudine, and add corticosteroids and possibly carnitine.

Immune reconstitution inflammatory syndrome (IRIS)

Conditions driven by CD4 lymphocytes (e.g. RA, SLE, and sarcoidosis) are rarely seen with HIV. Symptoms can regress with the development of HIV/AIDS and recur after treatment with HAART. This is termed immune reconstitution inflammatory syndrome (IRIS). In addition, new-onset RA, SLE, and sarcoidosis can occur in association with increasing CD4+ T-cell counts. During immune reconstitution there appears to be an increased risk of developing these symptoms above the pre-existing risk for that individual.

CD8+ driven conditions such as psoriasis, reactive arthritis, and DILS may be initial manifestations of HIV infection and should settle with HIV treatment.

Other opportunistic infections of muscle and bone may occur, especially atypical mycobacterial infections; *Mycobacterium haemophilum* and *Mycobacterium kansasii* are the two most frequent. Mycobacterium tuberculosis is no more frequent in HIV AIDS, but may emerge during immune reconstitution.

Disseminated histoplasmosis, cryptococcosis, sporotrichosis, and blastomycosis, leading to osteomyelitis, septic arthritis, or bursitis may also occur.

Avascular necrosis is seen in 3–5% of HIV patients. The hips are most commonly affected, but more than three joints are involved in 70% of affected patients. Possible contributory risk factors, in addition to HIV itself, are hyperlipidaemia, alcohol excess, use of high-dose steroids, and a hypercoagulable state. There may be an association with the use of HAART.

The whole spectrum of vasculitis has been reported, from small-vessel vasculitis to aortitis. Vasculitis has been described in early stage HIV when patients have preserved CD4 counts, as well as later in patients with severe immunosuppression. Patients commonly present with rash and peripheral neuropathy. HIV-associated cryoglobulinaemia, polyarteritis nodosa (PAN), and large-vessel complications such as strokes have been reported.

Osteoporosis

There are a number of reasons why patients with HIV are at increased risk of low bone mass. HAART treatment itself may contribute to low bone mass. In addition, HIV patients suffer from anorexia with associated vitamin D insufficiency, reduced lean body mass, and limited weight-bearing exercise. Smoking and excessive alcohol consumption is more common in HIV-infected patients.

Further reading

Medina Rodriguez F (2003). Rheumatic manifestations of human immunodeficiency virus. *Rheum Dis Clin North Am*; **29**: 145–61.

Plate A-M, Boyle B (2003). Musculoskeletal manifestations of HIV infection. *AIDS Read*; **13**: 62, 69–70, 72, 76.

Case 20

A 3-year-old Caucasian girl was referred to a paediatric rheumatology clinic with a 6-month history of a swollen right knee. She had not complained of any pain but her parents had noticed that she had stopped jumping on her trampoline. She had no history of injury. She was apyrexial and had no rashes. Her knee was warm with a boggy swelling and a reduced range of movement. The other joints and spine were normal. Slit-lamp ophthalmic assessment is shown in Fig. 20.1.

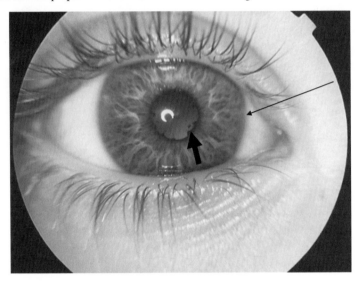

Fig. 20.1 (See also Plate 10) Slit-lamp examination of eye.

Questions

1. What is the differential diagnosis of a swollen joint in a child?
2. What further investigations would be helpful?
3. What is the most likely diagnosis?
4. What do the arrows in Fig. 20.1 indicate? What is the significance of the ophthalmologist's findings?
5. How would you manage this case?

Answers

1. What is the differential diagnosis of a swollen joint in a child?

The differential includes the following:

- Septic arthritis including chronic infection (e.g. tuberculosis)
- Trauma including non-accidental injury:
- Malignancy:
  - leukaemia
  - primary bone tumour
- JIA
- Haematological causes:
  - haemophilia (in a boy)
- Internal structural abnormalities:
  - discoid meniscus (knee)
  - osteochondritis dissecans
- Sarcoidosis (rare)
- Villonodular synovitis (rare).

2. What further investigations would be helpful?

Investigations in a young child should be performed where necessary but without causing undue distress. In this case they may include the following:

- FBC and blood film
- Inflammatory markers (e.g. CRP)
- ANA
- CXR if TB, sarcoid, or lymphoma are possibilities
- Ultrasound scan of the affected joint
- MRI scan of the affected joint
- Examination of joint aspirate
- ASOT if recent sore throat
- ELISPOT or QuantiFERON® if at risk of tuberculosis.

The FBC and inflammatory markers were normal and ANA was positive. An ultrasound scan of the knee demonstrated synovitis and an effusion. Inflammatory synovial fluid was aspirated under general anaesthesia and there was no evidence of infection.

3. What is the most likely diagnosis?

This child had oligoarticular disease and was systemically well. The presence of fever, severe pain, weight loss, or abnormalities of the blood film would raise concerns about malignancy or chronic infection which were unlikely in this case. The risk of tuberculosis was low. More detailed imaging with MRI would be indicated if bone tumour or intra-articular structural abnormalities were suspected on clinical grounds.

Ultrasound demonstration of synovitis with a good response to intra-articular steroid injection supported a diagnosis of JIA. Tests for ANA are positive in up to 85% of children with oligoarthritis, especially in girls and those children with uveitis. FBC and inflammatory markers are generally normal but may show signs of inflammation. Rheumatoid factor is not a useful test as it is almost always negative. A biopsy may be considered if sarcoid, villonodular synovitis, or chronic infection were suspected, or if there was an inadequate response to intra-articular steroids, leading to review of the diagnosis.

JIA is a chronic inflammatory disease beginning before the 16th birthday. The prevalence in the UK is 65 in 100 000 and the annual incidence is 10 in 100 000. Arthritis in children is different from that in adults both clinically and in pathogenesis. The different types of JIA (Table 20.1) can occur in any age group, but tend to peak at certain ages. Oligoarticular JIA tends to occur in toddlers and is associated with inflammatory eye disease. The child is usually systemically well.

A child has oligoarticular JIA if four or fewer joints are affected during the first 6 months of the disease. If more joints become affected, it is termed extended oligoarticular JIA. Generally the joints affected are lower limb; knee, ankle, and midfoot. Leg-length difference may result from increased bone growth around an affected knee relative to the normal side. Mid-foot and subtalar joint involvement may cause an everted foot posture and a smaller foot.

The peak incidence is between 2 and 4 years old, and it is more common in girls than boys with a female-to-male ratio of 3:1. The aetiology is poorly understood. Genome-wide studies have identified JIA susceptibility loci in the HLA region involved in T-cell receptor signalling and activation pathways.

4. What do the arrows in Fig. 20.1 indicate? What is the significance of the ophthalmologist's findings?

Slit-lamp examination showed early band-shaped keratopathy of the cornea (thin arrow), flare, cells in the anterior chamber, and synechiae (thick arrow) between the iris margin and the lens. Intra-ocular pressures were measured at a later date when full cooperation had been achieved and were found to be in the normal range. There was no posterior segment disease. The opthalmologist's findings were consistent with a diagnosis of anterior uveitis in keeping with JIA.

Table 20.1 International League of Associations for Rheumatology (ILAR) classification of juvenile idiopathic arthritis 2004

Category	Features
Oligoarthritis: ◆ Persistent ◆ Extended	Arthritis in 4 or fewer joints during the first 6 months of disease ◆ Never more than 4 affected joints ◆ More than 4 joints affected after the first 6 months *Exclusions 1, 2, 3, 4, 5*
Polyarthritis (rheumatoid factor positive)	Arthritis affecting 5 or more joints during the first 6 months of disease RF test is positive *Exclusions 1, 2, 3, 5*
Polyarthritis (rheumatoid factor negative)	Arthritis affecting 5 or more joints during the first 6 months of disease RF test is negative *Exclusions 1, 2, 3, 4, 5*
Systemic arthritis	Arthritis in any number of joints with fever of at least 2 weeks' duration, documented to be quotidian for at least 3 days, accompanied by one or more of: ◆ Evanescent rash ◆ Generalized lymphadenopathy ◆ Enlargement of liver or spleen ◆ Serositis *Exclusions 1, 2, 3, 4*
Psoriatic arthritis	Arthritis and psoriasis, or arthritis and at least 2 of: ◆ Dactylitis ◆ Nail pitting or onycholysis ◆ Psoriasis in first-degree relative *Exclusions 2, 3, 4, 5*
Enthesitis-related arthritis	Arthritis and enthesitis, or arthritis or enthesitis with at least 2 of: ◆ Sacroiliac joint tenderness and/or inflammatory lumbosacral pain ◆ The presence of HLA-B27 antigen ◆ Onset of arthritis in boy >6 years old ◆ Anterior uveitis (symptomatic) ◆ Family history of HLA-B27 associated disease *Exclusions 1, 4, 5*
Undifferentiated arthritis	◆ Fits no other category ◆ Fits more than one category
Exclusions	1. Psoriasis or a history of psoriasis in the patient or a first-degree relative. 2. Arthritis in an HLA-B27 positive male after the 6th birthday. 3. Ankylosing spondylitis, enthesitis-related arthritis, sacro-iliitis with IBD, reactive arthritis, or acute anterior uveitis or a history of one of these disorders in a first-degree relative. 4. The presence of IgM RF on at least 2 occasions, at least 3 months apart. 5. The presence of systemic JIA in the patient.

Uveitis is caused by inflammation in the anterior chamber of the eye and occurs in up to 20% of children with oligoarticular JIA. Inflammatory eye disease associated with JIA is the most common cause of chronic anterior uveitis in childhood and usually occurs in the oligoarticular subset. Uveitis is usually asymptomatic in children under 12 years old, and new-onset inflammatory eye disease rarely presents over this age. Although uveitis is five times more common in girls, boys are more likely to have severe disease.

A child may present with uveitis at the time of diagnosis and up to 7 years later, but eye inflammation precedes joint disease in 5% of cases. The severity of uveitis at presentation is a major factor in determining its outcome and in 70–80% cases is bilateral. A positive ANA is a risk factor in children, but those who have uveitis with a negative ANA are more likely to have severe disease. Regular screening is essential, and protocols are available depending on the type of arthritis and age of onset. Children under the age of 8 years have a particularly high risk of developing severe eye disease and should be very closely monitored for the first 2 years after diagnosis of JIA. Complications include cataract formation, glaucoma, and cystoid macular oedema, all of which are sight threatening. Amblyopia (lazy eye) can develop with even mild disease in children under 7. Band keratopathy is caused by calcium deposition in the cornea and is evidence of inflammation.

5. How would you manage this case?

Both disease course and management of eye and joint disease may differ in the same patient. The aim of management of JIA is to control synovitis, restore muscle strength, and encourage normal growth and movement. A multidisciplinary approach is required, including rheumatology, opthalmology, physiotherapy, occupational therapy, orthotics, and psychology.

Medications that may be used include the following:

- NSAIDs such as ibuprofen 30 mg/kg/day or diclofenac 1–3 mg/kg/day in divided doses provide symptomatic relief.
- Intra-articular joint injections with triamcinolone hexacetonide 1 mg/kg per joint. In young children this should be under a general anaesthetic and in older children the use of Entonox may help.
- Methotrexate is used when joint inflammation recurs despite intra-articular injection. This is prescribed orally or as subcutaneous injections at 15–20 mg/m^2/week.
- Children with five or more swollen joints and three or more joints with limitation of movement who have not responded to subcutaneous methotrexate 20 mg/m^2 may be considered for anti-TNF therapy.

Steroid eye drops are the mainstay of treatment of uveitis and can be instilled up to two-hourly in the first instance. The frequency should be slowly tapered over several months as the inflammation subsides. Short-acting cycloplegic (dilating) drops should also be applied to prevent progression of synechiae. Periocular injection of steroid under general anaesthetic is an option for severe or non-responsive cases.

Treatment with oral or subcutaneous methotrexate is considered when uveitis is uncontrolled by these measures. Ciclosporin, azathioprine, mycophenolate mofetil, and leflunomide may also be effective. The results from anti-TNF treatment are conflicting, but infliximab and adalimumab may be effective.

This patient was managed with intra-articular steroid injections under general anaesthetic, physiotherapy, and hydrotherapy. Her joint disease was rapidly controlled by steroid injection. The eye disease was initially treated with dexamethasone and 1% cyclopentalate drops but did not show a significant response. After 6 months she had developed severe bilateral anterior uveitis. Methotrexate therapy was commenced and the uveitis settled. Screening every 2–3 months will continue during childhood and monitoring will continue for life. She found the routine blood monitoring for methotrexate very upsetting and the help of the team psychologist was enlisted to support the family with strategies to reduce her distress.

Further reading

Cassidy JT, Petty RE (2005). *Textbook of Paediatric Rheumatology* (5th edn). Philadelphia, PA: Elsevier Saunders.

Edelsten C (2007). Reconsidering treatment options in childhood uveitis. *Br J Ophthalmol*; **91**: 133–4.

Edelsten C, Lee V, Bentley CR, Kanski JJ Graham EM (2002). An evaluation of baseline risk factors predicting severity in juvenile idiopathic arthritis associated uveitis and other chronic anterior uveitis in early childhood. *Br J Ophthalmol*; **86**: 51–6.

Petty RE, Southwood TR, Manners P, *et al.* (2004). International League of Associations for Rheumatology classification of juvenile idiopathic arthritis: second revision, Edmonton, 2001. *J Rheumatol*; **31**: 390–2.

Ravelli A, Martini A (2007). Juvenile idiopathic arthritis. *Lancet*; **369**: 767–78.

Case 21

A 19-year-old male with a history of recurrent fractures from birth was seen in the rheumatology department. He had sustained more than 40 fractures leading to painful skeletal deformity and he had been wheelchair-bound from the age of 10 years. His father was also affected by 'brittle bones' and was restricted to a wheelchair.

He was treated with cyclical intravenous pamidronate from the age of 10 years, which resulted in reduced bone pain. A baseline DEXA scan at age 14 years showed a T-score of −7.0 SD below the mean at the lumbar spine, which increased to −5.1 after 4 years of therapy (osteoporosis is defined as a T-score less than −2.5 SD below the mean for peak age). The infusions were discontinued at age 17 years when his family moved district. He developed increasing back and limb pain, which he attributed to cessation of the bisphosphonate, and required regular opiates and baclofen. He also reported troublesome morning headaches.

On examination, he was below the third centile for height with a severe thoracolumbar scoliosis. His teeth were translucent, with scalloped borders. His sclerae appeared normal. There was no objective muscle weakness.

Questions

1. What is the most likely diagnosis?
2. What is the pathogenesis?
3. What are the common clinical manifestations?
4. What investigations may be useful?
5. How would you manage this patient? Why might he have morning headache?

Answers

1. What is the most likely diagnosis and what is the classification?

The most likely diagnosis is osteogenesis imperfecta type III.

Osteogenesis imperfecta (OI) is a genetic condition characterized by bone fragility. This patient has OI type III on the basis of the autosomal dominant inheritance, severe disease resulting in multiple fractures at birth, progressive deformity through childhood, and short stature. Extra-skeletal manifestations include abnormal dentition (dentinogenesis imperfecta), but the sclera may appear normal (Table 21.1).

Currently, eight subtypes of OI are recognized (Table 21.1). Types I–IV are based on the Sillence clinical classification and are due to mutations in type I collagen genes (COL1A1 or COL1A2) with autosomal dominant inheritance. Affected individuals may have extra-skeletal manifestations. Type I is the most common subtype and may result in mild disease, type II is lethal in the perinatal period, and types III and IV range from moderate to severe.

The Sillence classification has been extended to include types V–VIII, which are phenotypically severe and lack extra-articular manifestations. Types VII and VIII are recessively inherited, and are due to genetic mutations affecting proteins involved in post-translational processing of type I collagen (CRTAP/LEPRE genes). The genetic bases of types V and VI have yet to be fully characterized.

2. What is the pathogenesis?

Most cases of OI are due to gene mutations in type I collagen which is the predominant collagen component of the bony organic matrix. Type I collagen is composed of a triple helix of polypeptide chains, with glycine positioned regularly within the peptide sequence cross-linking the chains together.

Two major genetic mechanisms are responsible for bone fragility in OI.

◆ Milder disease (particularly OI type I) may be due to an extra stop codon or frameshift mutation within the type I collagen gene. The abnormally truncated polypeptide chains are removed by the cell and are not incorporated into the triple helix. As the condition is autosomal dominant, some normal polypeptides are formed and the patient is left with reduced production of normal collagen helices.

◆ In OI types II–IV mutations typically code for amino acid substitutions of a glycine residue. This alters the stability of the triple helices by interfering with cross-linking between the normal and abnormal polypeptide chains. Severe disease may result if the affected glycine is at a crucial position.

3. What are the common clinical manifestations?

The defining characteristic of OI is bone fragility resulting in susceptibility to fracture. Although typically diagnosed in childhood, OI type I may be mild and therefore may present at any age. It is crucial to exclude non-accidental injury in a child presenting with recurrent fracture.

Extra-skeletal manifestations may be present in patients with OI types I–IV. These may be subtle and difficult to detect. They include the following:

- Blue sclera: the pigmented choroid is visible through an abnormally translucent sclera. This can be difficult to recognize as it is relatively common in non-Caucasian children with or without OI.
- Dentinogenesis imperfecta ('shell teeth'): discoloured translucent teeth which are susceptible to damage resulting in scalloped borders.
- Conductive hearing loss: this is due to fractures and subsequent fibrosis of the ossicles of the middle ear. Hearing impairment is particularly common in adults over the age of 50 years.

4. What investigations may be useful?

In the presence of a positive family history of fracture and typical extra-skeletal manifestations such as blue sclera or dentinogenesis imperfecta, no further investigations are required. However, in equivocal cases the following may be helpful.

- X-ray: although not pathognomonic, a mosaic appearance on skull X-ray may be seen due to numerous wormian bones. Wormian bones are irregular bony plates that form between the cranial sutures.
- Limb X-ray: a hypertrophic callus or calcified forearm interosseous membrane may indicate OI type V. OI types VII and VIII may be indicated by 'popcorn epiphyses'.
- DEXA scan: bone density is reduced.
- Genetics/proteomics: samples of serum or saliva can be collected and screened for mutations in the type I collagen or CRTAP/LEPRE genes (Table 21.1). Alternatively, fibroblasts isolated from a skin biopsy can be cultured and assessed for the quantity and quality of type I procollagen protein. Approximately 90% of cases affecting collagen type I genes can be detected by these methods (OI types I–IV). However, they are less helpful for OI subgroups V–VIII.
- Bone biopsy: in most cases, biopsy will show a reduced cortical thickness of bone in association with reduced trabecular density and size. This is an invasive test but may be diagnostic, particularly in OI types V and VI (Table 21.1).

5. How would you manage this patient?

Management of severe cases should be coordinated in a specialist centre. Treatment includes physiotherapy, rehabilitation, orthotics, and surgery to minimize disability. Bisphosphonates may improve bone density, mobility, and grip strength, and reduce the incidence of fracture and bone pain. Treatment in severe OI is most effective when given in the growth phase, and cyclical intravenous pamidronate is the most commonly used regimen in children. The long-term safety of bisphosphonate therapy in children is unclear, and there may be theoretical risks of impaired postoperative bone healing. In the longer term there is also concern about prior pamidronate administration in women of childbearing age which may reduce the availability of skeletal calcium for fetal bone formation.

This patient should probably re-start bisphosphonate therapy. Options include regular intravenous pamidronate or zoledronate. Alternatively, as an adult, he may tolerate oral preparations such as alendronic acid or risedronate. It is essential to ensure an adequate intake of calcium and vitamin D.

Management of the extra-skeletal manifestations of OI and monitoring for complications is important. This patient should be referred to a maxillofacial surgeon for optimal care of the dental abnormalities. Severe kyphoscoliosis may result in a restrictive respiratory deficit. The symptoms of morning headache may indicate nocturnal hypoventilation; a referral to the respiratory team would be warranted for consideration of nocturnal non-invasive ventilation.

Table 21.1 Classification of osteogenesis imperfecta

Type	Gene	Inheritance	Severity	Clinical features
I	Abnormal stop codon or frameshift mutation in COL1A1 or COL1A2 gene	AD	◆ Most common and mildest OI subtype ◆ Increased fracture risk ◆ Non-deforming ◆ May present at any age including elderly	◆ Normal height ◆ Minimal deformity ◆ Vertebral wedge fractures common especially in puberty ◆ Blue sclera
II	Typically due to point mutations in COL1A1 or COL1A2	AD	◆ Lethal perinatally due to multiple fractures and respiratory complications	◆ Multiple fractures at birth ◆ Grey sclera ◆ Wormian bones on skull X-ray
III		AD	◆ Severe ◆ Wheelchair-bound ◆ Progressive deformity throughout childhood ◆ Respiratory compromise	◆ Multiple fractures at birth ◆ Short stature ◆ White/grey sclera ◆ Severe dentinogenesis imperfecta ◆ Triangular facies ◆ Early hearing loss ◆ Wormian bones on skull X-ray
IV		AD	◆ Moderate to severe ◆ Progressive deformity throughout childhood	◆ Moderate short stature ◆ Dentinogenesis imperfecta ◆ Early hearing loss

Table 21.1 (*Contd.*)

Type	Gene	Inheritance	Severity	Clinical features
V	Not characterized	AD	◆ Moderate to severe	◆ Moderate short stature ◆ Calcified interroseous membrane causing radial head dislocation ◆ Hypertrophic callus after fracture ◆ Mesh-like appearance of bone lamellae histologically
VI	Not characterized	AR	◆ Moderate to severe	◆ Moderate short stature ◆ Scoliosis ◆ Fish-scale appearance of bone lamellae and increased osteoid histologically
VII	Reduced expression of cartilage-associated protein (CRTAP) involved in post-translational modification of collagen type I	AR	◆ Moderate to severe	◆ Mild short stature ◆ Limb length discrepancy ◆ Coxa vara ◆ 'Popcorn epiphyses'
VIII	Mutations in prolyl-3-hydroxylase-1 (LEPRE1) involved in post-translational modification of collagen type I	AR	◆ Severe	◆ Marked short stature ◆ Reduced mineralization of fractures ◆ Barrel-shaped chest ◆ 'Popcorn epiphyses'

AD: autosomal dominant; AR: autosomal recessive. Data from Basel D, Steiner RD (2009). Osteogenesis imperfecta: recent findings shed new light on this once well-understood condition. *Genet Med*; **11**: 375–85.

Further reading

Basel D, Steiner RD (2009). Osteogenesis imperfecta: recent findings shed new light on this once well-understood condition. *Genet Med*; **11**: 375–85.

Cheung MS, Glorieux FH (2008). Osteogenesis Imperfecta: update on presentation and management. *Rev Endocr Metab Disord*; **9**: 153–60.

Phillipi CA, Remmington T, Steiner RD (2008). Bisphosphonate therapy for osteogenesis imperfecta. *Cochrane Database Syst Rev*; **8**: CD005088.

Case 22

A 25-year-old male presented with a 4-week history of right anterior shin pain. He was an office worker who had recently commenced running regularly in order to compete in the London Marathon for a charitable organization. The marathon was 3 months away. He had been a competitive long-distance runner as a teenager, but had led a sedentary lifestyle in recent years.

His symptoms had initially been a mild ache in his right anterior shin towards the end of a 10 mile run, but this had gradually worsened over the past 2 weeks to the point where he now had pain with any weight-bearing activity and was unable to run. There was occasional night pain. He had tried paracetamol and NSAIDs but had received no symptomatic benefit.

Examination revealed an antalgic gait. He was unable to hop on the right leg because of pain. There was point tenderness and subtle swelling over a 3cm region in the distal third of the tibia on the medial aspect. He had weak hip abductors and poor core stability.

A plain radiograph of his right tibia was normal.

Questions

1. What is the differential diagnosis?
2. How would you manage this patient acutely?
3. What further imaging would you do to help clarify the diagnosis?
4. Are there any other investigations that may be useful?
5. What advice should you give him regarding returning to running?
6. Will he be able to compete in the marathon?

Answers

1. What is the differential diagnosis?

The differential diagnoses in order of probability in this patient are as follows.

- Tibial stress fracture: the inability to hop (especially if this is due to impact pain) and the point tenderness suggest the diagnosis of a stress fracture.

- Medial tibial stress syndrome (MTSS): this remains a strong possibility. MTSS is due to a traction periostitis where tendons attach to the tibia and is the most common cause of anterior shin pain. It commonly occurs in runners who suddenly increase their frequency or intensity of training, or who use worn-out shoes. Swelling and tenderness over the distal portion of the tibia are consistent with this diagnosis. Pain with resisted plantar flexion could be the reason for the inability to hop.

- Chronic exercise-induced anterior compartment syndrome: this diagnosis is very unlikely in the current scenario, but is listed here because it is a differential diagnosis of shin pain. Patients with chronic exercise-induced compartment syndrome do not usually present acutely and do not usually have point tenderness or impact pain. Common symptoms are anterolateral shin pain of gradual onset that becomes progressively worse with exercise and improves within a few minutes of rest. There may be exercise-associated foot drop, or sensory symptoms in the distribution of the deep peroneal nerve.

- Osteoid osteoma: the limited night pain and lack of response to anti-inflammatories are against the diagnosis of osteoid osteoma, but it should be considered in this age group, especially if night pain were a major feature. Osteoid osteomas are small (<2 cm) benign prostaglandin-producing tumours that can occur in any bone, but the femur and tibia are the most common sites. Males under the age of 30 are the highest risk group. Prostaglandin production by the tumour causes local bone pain which is responsive to anti-inflammatory medication.

2. How would you manage this patient acutely?

The working diagnosis is tibial stress fracture. The initial management is to make the patient non-weight-bearing. Options would be to put on an Aircast® boot or plaster of Paris and provide him with crutches. He should be encouraged to do non-weight-bearing exercise, such as swimming, to maintain his fitness and muscle tone. This is called 'relative rest'. A decision on how long he should be non-weight-bearing will depend on imaging results and improvement in symptoms.

3. What further imaging would you do to help clarify the diagnosis?

There are three options for imaging.

- ◆ MRI is the imaging option of choice. MRI will usually be able to identify bone stress, demonstrate fracture lines, identify areas of periosteal reaction and soft tissue pathology.

- ◆ Nuclear bone scan will show a hot spot in the context of a stress fracture, increased bone turnover, or a periosteal reaction. Bone scans are good at identifying the presence of abnormal pathology, but not at discriminating the aetiology of the underlying problem. A positive bone scan will need to be followed up with a CT of the abnormal area.

- ◆ A CT scan will evaluate the bony architecture and therefore demonstrate a cortical breach, fracture lines, cortical thickening due to new bone formation (Fig. 22.1), or a 'nidus' in the case of an osteoid osteoma. The main drawbacks of CT are the limited soft tissue information and the radiation dose.

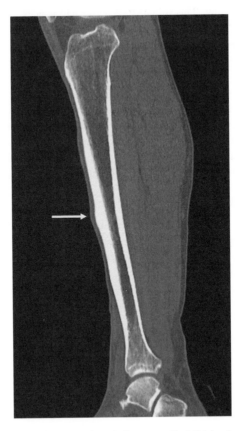

Fig. 22.1 CT scan of tibia. The arrow is pointing to cortical thickening of the anterior tibia. This is consistent with bone stress or a healing stress fracture.

4. Are there any other investigations that may be useful?

Vitamin D levels should be checked, and replaced if low. A large proportion of patients presenting with stress fractures are vitamin D deficient. It is uncertain whether low vitamin D directly contributes to the development of stress fracture or if it is simply an observed association. In a female patient the female athlete triad of amenorrhea, anorexia, and osteoporosis should be considered and appropriately managed. The weak hip abduction may be part of the vitamin D deficiency. Physiotherapy will be helpful in addressing this when he has replenished his stores.

5. What advice should you give him regarding returning to running?

A tibial stress fracture requires the patient to be non-weight-bearing for 2–4 weeks and in a boot for approximately 4 weeks. Partial, followed by full, weight-bearing will be guided by symptoms and clinical improvement. Clinical improvement is gauged by the ability to hop pain free on the affected leg and resolution of tibial tenderness. Once fully weight-bearing, return to running will need to be done in a slow stepwise manner. This should start with a gentle walk–jog programme, with the intensity and duration of jogging slowly increasing over a period of months. Any biomechanical abnormalities which may have contributed to the stress fracture such as over-pronation, weak hip abductors, and poor core stability should be addressed.

This man had a tibial stress fracture which was demonstrated on MRI scan. The area of bone stress correlated with his local pain on the medial aspect of the distal third of the tibia. His 25OH-vitamin D levels were 15 nmol/L, which is low. He was given 50 000 IU of vitamin D daily for 7 days and thereafter one capsule per week for 6 weeks. He worked with the physiotherapist, and his pain resolved in 8 weeks and his muscle power returned to normal after 4 months.

6. Will he be able to compete in the marathon?

No, he will not be able to compete in a marathon in 3 months. He should be advised that he will need a much longer period to increase his running distance and intensity slowly in order to compete safely. He could aim to compete in the London Marathon the following year.

Case 23

A 51-year-old man presented with a 2-day history of increasing exertional breathlessness and cough productive of a moderate amount of fresh blood. Over the preceding 3 weeks he had felt very fatigued and noticed migratory joint and muscle pains. On further enquiry, he had seen his GP several times in the last year for a recurrent blocked nose which had been treated as allergic sinusitis. In the past month his nasal symptoms had changed to a foul-smelling discharge. He had no significant past medical history.

On examination he had a fever of 37.9°C, blood pressure of 160/100 mmHg, and O_2 saturations of 89% on air. There was diffuse nasal mucosal swelling and redness with some areas of ulceration and crusting. Bronchial breath sounds were heard in the mid and lower zones of both lung fields. Neurological examination revealed conductive hearing loss in his left ear. The remainder of the cardiovascular system, gastrointestinal, and musculoskeletal examination was normal.

Investigations showed the following:

- Hb 9.4 g/dL; WCC 13.2 × 10⁹/mL; neutrophils 9.1 × 10⁹/mL; platelets 623 × 10⁹/L
- Serum creatinine 488 μmol/L
- Urea 32 mmol/L
- CRP >160 mg/L
- CXR—see Fig. 23.1
- Urine microscopy: red cell casts present.

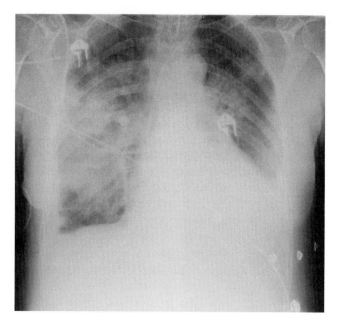

Fig. 23.1 CXR showing pulmonary haemorrhage.

Questions

1. What is the differential diagnosis?
2. What tests will help to differentiate between the possible diagnoses?
3. How should this man be managed in the acute setting?
4. What is his prognosis?
5. What can be done to reduce the risk of relapse?

Answers

1. What is the differential diagnosis?

The differential diagnosis includes the pulmonary renal syndromes.

Red cell casts in the urine indicate glomerular damage. The most common cause of glomerular damage is glomerular inflammation but other causes include renal infarction and bacterial endocarditis. The elevated serum creatinine and hypertension support severe renal involvement. The CXR showed bilateral air space opacity with some apical sparing. Diffuse pulmonary haemorrhage is the most likely cause of the CXR findings. Infection is less likely because it is bilateral, but needs to be excluded. The main differentials for a pulmonary renal syndrome are as follows.

◆ Wegener's granulomatosis (WG): WG is a necrotizing vasculitis of small and medium-sized blood vessels in which granulomatous inflammation of the respiratory tract occurs. The newer nomenclature for this condition is granulomatosis with polyangiitis (GPA). Lung capillaritis, which can result in pulmonary haemorrhage and necrotizing glomerulonephritis, is a common feature.

◆ Microscopic polyangiitis (MPA): MPA is a necrotizing vasculitis with few or no immune deposits, predominantly affecting small-calibre vessels. Necrotizing glomerulonephritis and pulmonary haemorrhage from capillaritis are the characteristic features. The lack of granulomatous inflammation of the respiratory tract is the main distinguishing clinical feature between MPA and WG.

◆ Goodpasture's syndrome (anti-glomerular basement membrane disease): This is a rare autoimmune condition where antibodies against the α3-subunit of type IV collagen found in the lung and kidney cause pulmonary haemorrhage and glomerulonephritis.

◆ Systemic lupus erythematosus (SLE): SLE is an autoimmune connective tissue disease with a wide spectrum of presentations including multisystem disease involving the lung and kidney. It typically affects women between the ages of 15 and 50 years.

The history of nasal congestion, crusting, and conductive deafness favours a diagnosis of WG. These items are not typical features of the other differential diagnoses, and the patient's gender and age make SLE unlikely.

2. What tests will help to differentiate between the possible diagnoses?

◆ Anti-neutrophil cytoplasm antibodies (ANCA) are present in most patients with WG and MPA and are helpful in confirming the diagnosis in the appropriate clinical context. However, they should not be used as a screening test. ANCA can be detected in two ways.

• Indirect immunofluorescence assay to identify specific staining patterns on human neutrophils by the antibodies. A cytoplasmic (c-ANCA) staining pattern is observed in most patients with WG, whereas a perinuclear pattern (p-ANCA) is seen with MPA (Fig. 23.2).

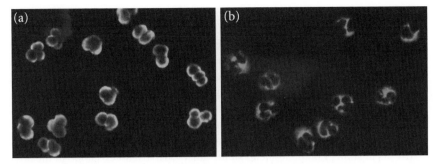

Fig. 23.2 (See also Plate 11). Antineutrophil cytoplasm antibodies as seen with indirect immunofluorescence: (a) perinuclear staining pattern (p-ANCA); (b) cytoplasmic staining pattern (c-ANCA).

Source: private collection of Raashid Luqmani.

- Enzyme-linked immunosorbent assay (ELISA). Antibody directed against proteinase 3 (PR3) is strongly associated with WG (and c-ANCA). Antibodies against myeloperoxidase (MPO) are associated with MPA (and p-ANCA), but can also be found in other vasculitic syndromes and IBD.

♦ Anti-glomerular basement membrane (GBM) antibodies are diagnostic of Goodpasture's syndrome. ANCA tests can be positive in around 20% of patients with Goodpasture's syndrome and in those patients there is a more favourable prognosis.

♦ Anti nuclear antibody (ANA) tests can be performed to rule out a diagnosis of SLE. Over 95% of patients with SLE will have a positive ANA, but the test is not specific for the diagnosis. In this clinical setting, a negative test would be helpful.

♦ Nasal mucosal biopsy showing necrotizing granulomatous vasculitis is strongly suggestive of WG.

♦ Renal biopsy: all the differential diagnoses mentioned above may show evidence of a rapidly progressive crescentic glomerulonephritis on histology. IgG deposits visible along the glomerular basement membrane on microscopy with immunofluorescence staining is suggestive of Goodpasture's syndrome. Immune complexes directed against immunoglobulins or complement can be seen in patients with lupus nephritis.

♦ Other tissue biopsies such as lung or nerve may be useful in different settings, but the above-mentioned tests should be sufficient to make the diagnosis in this patient.

3. How should this man be managed in the acute setting?

This patient has organ- and life-threatening disease as demonstrated by diffuse alveolar haemorrhage and renal failure. He is probably best managed in an intensive care unit/high-dependency unit where his respiratory function can be closely monitored and mechanical ventilation can be provided if required. Treatment includes plasma exchange (to remove circulating autoantibodies and immune complexes which may be driving this process) and immunosuppressive therapy with cyclophosphamide and glucocorticoids. The MEPEX trial showed that plasma exchange improved the renal outcome for patients with severe renal vasculitis. In addition, there is a consensus that plasma exchange should be used for pulmonary haemorrhage, with evidence from retrospective case series. However, randomized trial evidence is not yet available. Intravenous pulse cyclophosphamide at a dose of 15 mg/kg every 3 weeks is given for up to 6 months in conjunction with oral prednisolone at a dose of 1 mg/kg daily (the dose of steroid is slowly tapered). Intravenous cyclophosphamide is favoured over continuous oral cyclophosphamide as it has similar efficacy but lower cumulative dose and thus lower long-term toxicity. This treatment strategy is applicable to all the differential diagnoses, although the dose of cyclophosphamide is usually lower (10 mg/kg) for SLE because of the higher risk of infective complications associated with this disease.

This patient was found to have a c-ANCA >160 IU. A diagnosis of WG was made. He was treated with 60 mg of prednisolone daily and given cyclophosphamide 1g intravenously every 3 weeks for six cycles. He was given co-trimoxazole 960 mg three times a week as pneumocystis prophylaxis and to reduce nasal carriage of *Staphylococcus aureus*, alendronate 70 mg weekly, and omeprazole 20 mg daily. His hypertension was treated with amlodipine. His renal function stabilized at creatinine 190 mmol/L by 3 months.

4. What is his prognosis?

The mortality rate for patients with a diagnosis of WG or MPA and renal failure at presentation is approximately 25% in the first year and highest in the first 3 months when the vasculitis is most active and immunosuppressive therapy is maximal. The mortality rate is even higher for patients requiring admission to an intensive care unit. The main causes of death are infection, pulmonary haemorrhage, and complications of severe renal failure. The risk of death is higher in those who remain dialysis-dependent than in those who regain renal function and are dialysis-independent. Those who do not regain renal function probably have severe disease and/or a delay in receiving appropriate therapy. If patients survive the initial 12 months, the prognosis improves, but there is increased long-term morbidity and mortality from the results of renal or other organ damage and increased risk of malignancy from cyclophosphamide exposure.

This patient had a relatively uneventful course. He had one episode of presumed pulmonary sepsis which was treated with antibiotics. He went onto mycophenolate mofetil 2 g daily after the cyclophosphamide therapy was completed at 22 weeks. His BP was treated with amlodipine and doxazocin.

5. What can be done to reduce the risk of relapse?

Once the disease activity is controlled with cyclophosphamide (i.e. the patient is in remission), treatment should be changed to less toxic immunosuppressive therapy. Azathioprine is the most common medication used for maintenance of remission and should be continued for a minimum of 18 months but often for up to 5 years. Other options for maintenance therapy are methotrexate, leflunomide, and mycophenolate mofetil. Earlier withdrawal of maintenance therapy is associated with a high rate of relapse. In addition, chronic nasal carriage of *Staph.aureus* has been associated with higher rates of relapse. Prophylactic use of co-trimoxazole may be useful in this setting. Prednisolone should ideally be tapered and stopped by the time maintenance therapy is commenced, but if this is not possible owing to persistent low-grade disease, it should be continued at the lowest possible dose. Patients with WG are at two- to threefold increased risk of cardiovascular morbidity, so modifiable risk factors such as smoking, dyslipidaemia, and hypertension should be addressed. Bone protection with calcium, vitamin D, and bisphosphonates should be considered in patients at increased risk of osteoporotic fracture, especially those who require ongoing glucocorticoid therapy, are post-menopausal, and/or have low baseline BMD.

Additional Reading

Jayne D, Rasmussen N, Andrassy K, *et al.* (2003). A randomized trial of maintenance therapy for vasculitis associated with antineutrophil cytoplasmic autoantibodies. *N Engl J Med*; **349**(1): p. 36–44.

Jayne DR, Gaskin G, Rasmussen N, *et al.* (2007). Randomized trial of plasma exchange or high-dosage methylprednisolone as adjunctive therapy for severe renal vasculitis. *J Am Soc Nephrol*; **18**: 2180–8.

Jennette JC, Falk RJ, Andrassy K, *et al.* (1994). Nomenclature of systemic vasculitides. Proposal of an international consensus conference. *Arthritis Rheum*; **37**: 187–92.

Hudson BG, Tryggvason K, Sundaramoorthy M, *et al.* (2003). Alport's syndrome, Goodpasture's syndrome, and type IV collagen. *N Engl J Med*; **348**: 2543–56.

Koldingsnes W, Nossent H (2002). Predictors of survival and organ damage in Wegener's granulomatosis. *Rheumatology*; **41**: 572–81.

Mukhtyar C, Flossmann O, Hellmich B, *et al.* (2008). Outcomes from studies of antineutrophil cytoplasm antibody associated vasculitis: a systematic review by the European League Against Rheumatism systemic vasculitis task force. *Ann Rheum Dis*; **67**: 1004–10.

Case 24

A 31-year-old woman presented to the rheumatology department with a 2-year history of arthralgia of her hands, wrists, and ankles, associated with early morning stiffness. Her past medical history included mild asthma and depression. She smoked 15 cigarettes a day. There was no family history of arthritis or autoimmune disease.

On examination, she had swelling of the small joints of her hands and wrists, with wasting of the intrinsic muscles and reduced grip strength. There was a small nodule at her left elbow. The CXR was unremarkable, and her hand X-rays suggested carpal crowding and periarticular osteopenia, with possible small erosion at the distal end of her proximal phalanx. The diagnosis of rheumatoid arthritis was made, and she was treated with intramuscular steroid, methotrexate, and hydroxychloroquine.

The following year, she presented with shortness of breath on exertion. Her methotrexate was stopped, but the shortness of breath progressed and she developed orthopnoea. On admission, she was found to be tachycardic and hypertensive. The CXR (Fig. 24.1) demonstrated an increase in the cardiac silhouette. An echocardiogram demonstrated a pericardial effusion, as well as a severely dilated left atrium, mitral regurgitation, and a reduced ejection fraction at 49%. An MRI gadolinium cardiac scan showed left ventricular hypertrophy, a dilated left atrium, a pericardial effusion, moderate mitral regurgitation, and a thrombus in the left apex. It also demonstrated endomyocardial inflammation or fibrosis (Fig. 24.2).

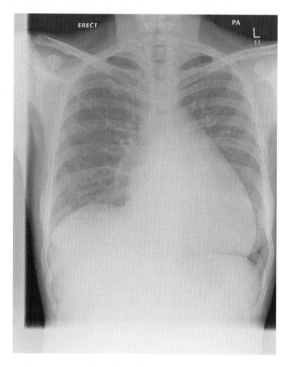

Fig. 24.1 CXR showing increased cardiac silhouette.

Questions

1. Give a differential diagnosis at her initial presentation with joint pains.

2. What are the current recommendations for management of rheumatoid arthritis (RA)?

3. What are the causes of shortness of breath in RA? Give a differential diagnosis based on the CXR findings.

4. What is the differential diagnosis for the endomyocardial inflammation or fibrosis?

5. What are the current NICE guidelines for starting biological therapy in RA?

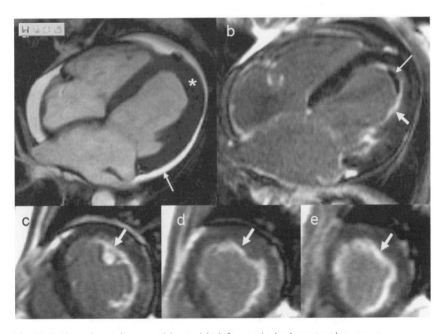

Fig. 24.2 The echocardiogram: (a) asterisk, left ventricular hypertrophy; arrow, pericardial effusion; (b) thin arrow, thrombus in apex; thick arrow, endomyocardial enhancement demonstrating inflammation or fibrosis; (c), (d), (e) arrows show the endomyocardial enhancement pattern.

The patient had a coronary angiogram which was normal, excluding an ischaemic cause. The patient was commenced on warfarin for the apical thrombus.

Her haematology data was reviewed and she was found to have an eosinophilia of 37% (normally <5%).

Oral corticosteroids were given and an infliximab infusion commenced because of ongoing high DAS and lack of efficacy of multiple DMARDs.

Answers

1. Give a differential diagnosis for the initial presentation of joint pains

The most likely diagnosis is nodular rheumatoid arthritis because there was a symmetrical small-joint polyarthritis with wrist involvement, wasting of the intrinsic muscles, and a nodule at the elbow. There is periarticular osteopenia on X-ray. These are consistent with a the diagnosis of RA.

Other causes of a polyarthritis include the following:

◆ Psoriatic arthritis

◆ Reactive arthritis

◆ Osteoarthritis

◆ Connective tissue disease (e.g. SLE)

◆ Vasculitis

◆ Sarcoidosis

◆ Malignancy (e.g. leukaemia).

These are less likely given the absence of other supporting features such as a rash, history of preceding infection, family history, erythema nodosum, or marked constitutional upset.

2. What are the current recommendations for management of rheumatoid arthritis?

The BSR guidelines for the management of new-onset disease suggest the following:

◆ Refer patients with suspected persistent synovitis of undetermined cause for specialist opinion. Patients should be offered ongoing access to the multidisciplinary team, including specialist physiotherapist and occupational therapist.

◆ Offer a combination of DMARDs, including methotrexate and at least one other DMARD, plus short-term glucocorticoids as first-line treatment as soon as possible.

◆ To monitor disease, use CRP and the key components of DAS.

The DAS is a combined index that was developed in Nijmegen in the 1980s to measure the disease activity in patients with RA. It has been validated for use in clinical trials in combination with the EULAR response criteria. There are DAS calculators that make it easy to use, and thus it is possible to collect information about the disease activity and response to treatment.

The DAS takes into account the number of swollen and tender joints, the ESR or CRP, and a Visual Analogue Score (VAS) of perceived patient disease activity. The score is between 0 and 10 and indicates how active the RA is at the time of measurement.

The DAS has been used to define thresholds for disease activity: high disease activity (>3.7); moderate (2.4<DAS<3.7); low (<2.4); remission (<1.6)

3. What are the causes of shortness of breath in RA? What does the CXR in Fig. 24.1 show? Give a differential diagnosis based on the CXR findings

The causes of shortness of breath in rheumatoid arthritis are as follows.

- Pulmonary:
  - non-specific interstitial pneumonia (NSIP)
  - idiosyncratic allergic alveolitis associated with drugs such as methotrexate, leflunomide, salazopyrine
  - pulmonary fibrosis
  - pleural effusion
  - pulmonary hypertension.

- Cardiac:
  - pericarditis
  - pericardial effusion
  - cardiac amyloid.

- Haematological:
  - anaemia.

The CXR demonstrates a significant increase in the cardiac silhouette size. The differential diagnosis of this includes:

- left ventricular failure
- pericardial effusion
- left ventricular hypertrophy
- dilated cardiomyopathy
- hypertrophic cardiomyopathy.

4. What is the differential diagnosis for the endomyocardial inflammation or fibrosis?

The differential diagnoses for the endomyocardial inflammation or fibrosis are:

- cardiac amyloid
- hypertensive heart disease
- ischaemic heart disease
- rare side effects of DMARDs
- eosinophilic myocarditis.

Other causes of myocarditis might include:

- infective (viral—adenovirus, parvovirus, human herpes virus 6, HIV)
- connective tissue disorders (e.g. SLE, scleroderma)
- sarcoidosis.

The pattern of endomyocardial enhancement seen on echocardiography in this case was considered to be typical of eosinophilic myocarditis rather than amyloidosis.

There is a documented association between RA and eosinophilia. This was first described in the 1970s. It was later recognized that there are two patterns of eosinophilia: one related to the disease process itself, and the other related to therapy (e.g. gold, penicillamine). The extra-articular features of RA, such as pericarditis, pulmonary fibrosis, and rheumatoid nodules, are more common in patients with eosinophilia. The relationship between tissue eosinophilia and RA is less well known. There are documented cases of RA with eosinophilic pneumonia, eosinophilic enteritis, and even eosinophilic meningoencephalitis, where no other cause for the eosinophilia is found.

Eosinophils are known to be harmful to the myocardium. Chronic eosinophilia has been associated with endomyocardial fibrosis and myocardial damage. This tissue injury is a direct result of degranulation of toxic eosinophilic granule proteins.

Other causes of eosinophilic myocarditis include

◆ idiopathic hypereosinophilia syndrome

◆ parasites

◆ rejected heart transplant

◆ drug reactions

◆ vasculitis (Churg–Strauss syndrome (CSS)).

The patient was successfully immunosuppressed with infliximab and this normalized her eosinophilic count. She showed improvement in her cardiac function, including a reduction in left ventricular mass, a rise in ejection fraction from 46% to 74%, and a reduction of the endomyocardial enhancement demonstrated previously.

5. What are the current NICE guidelines for starting biological therapy in RA?

The current NICE guidelines for starting biological therapy in RA are as follows (Table 24.1).

◆ The TNF-α inhibitors (adalimumab, etanercept and infliximab) are recommended as options for treatment in those with active RA as measured by the DAS, i.e. >5.1 on at least two occasions, or those who have undergone trials of two DMARDs (usually for a minimum of 6 months).

◆ Rituximab in combination with methotrexate is recommended as an option for the treatment of severe RA in those who have had an inadequate response or intolerance to other DMARDs, including treatment with at least one TNF-α inhibitor.

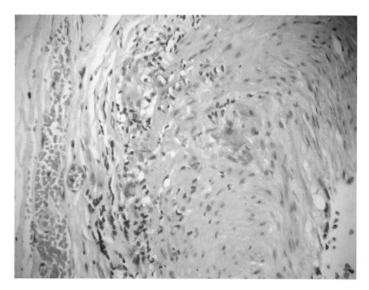

Plate 1 (See also Fig. 2.1) Diagnostic investigation.

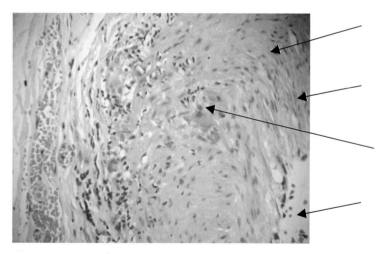

Plate 2 (See also Fig. 2.3) Temporal artery biopsy.

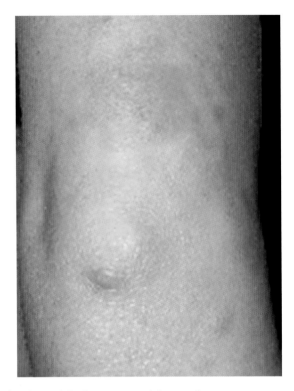

Plate 3 (See also Fig. 3.1) Erythematous nodules on elbow.

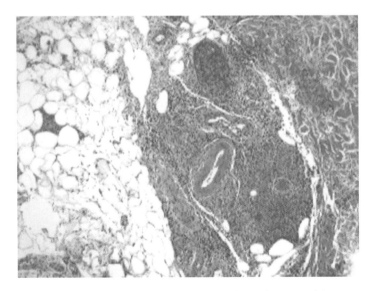

Plate 4 (See also Fig. 3.2) Skin biopsy with haematoxylin and eosin staining.

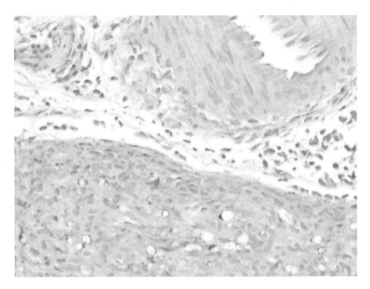

Plate 5 (See also Fig. 3.3) Skin biopsy with Wade–Fite staining.

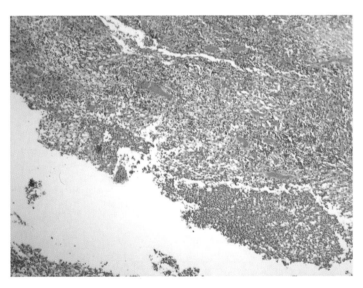

Plate 6 (See also Fig. 6.1) Linear fissuring ulcer formed by granulation tissue on either side, and containing neutrophils.

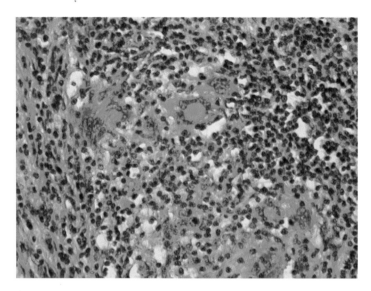

Plate 7 (See also Fig. 6.2) Granulomatous inflammation and giant cells.

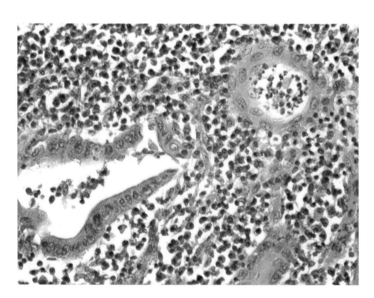

Plate 8 (See also Fig. 6.3) Distorted acutely inflamed colonic crypts (crypt abscesses).

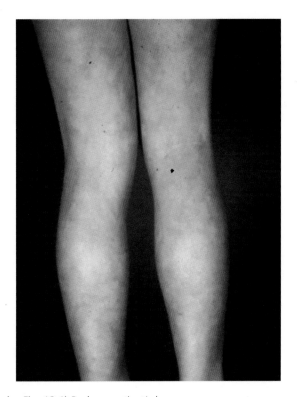

Plate 9 (See also Fig. 13.1) Rash on patient's legs.

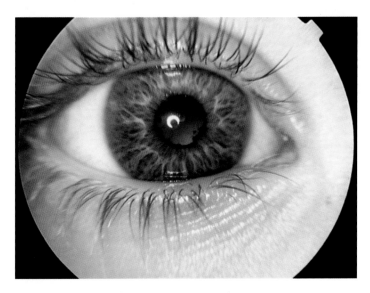

Plate 10 (See also Fig. 20.1) Slit-lamp examination of eye.

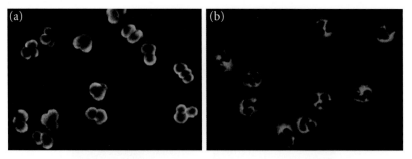

Plate 11 (See also Fig. 23.2) Antineutrophil cytoplasm antibodies as seen with indirect immunofluorescence: (a) perinuclear staining pattern (p-ANCA); (b) cytoplasmic staining pattern (c-ANCA).

Source: private collection of Raashid Luqmani.

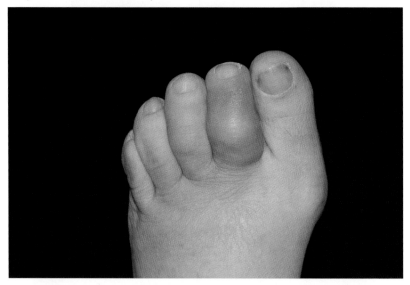

Plate 12 (See also Fig. 25.1) Dactylitis of left second toe.

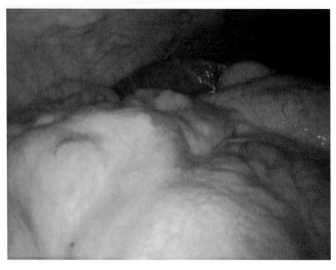

Plate 13 (See also Fig. 30.1) Mass of lymph nodes in the mesentery of the small bowel.

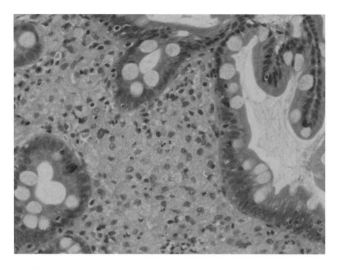

Plate 14 (See also Fig. 30.2) Photomicrographs of the duodenal biopsy showing macrophages containing PAS-positive granules.

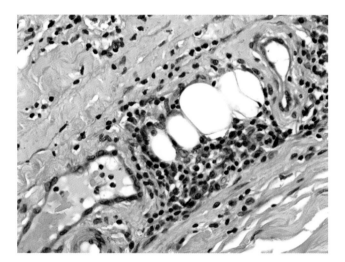

Plate 15 (See also Fig. 35.1) Fascial sclerosis with lymphocytic, plasma cell, and eosinophilic infiltration. (Reproduced from Servy A *et al.* (2010) *Patholog Res Int* © 2011 Amandine Servy *et al.*)

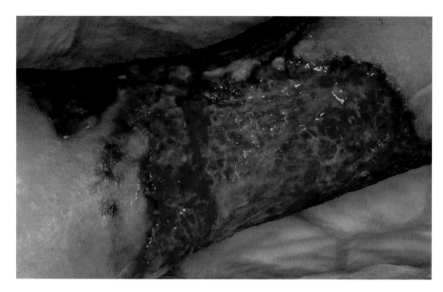

Plate 16 (See also Fig. 36.1) Circumferential leg ulcer.

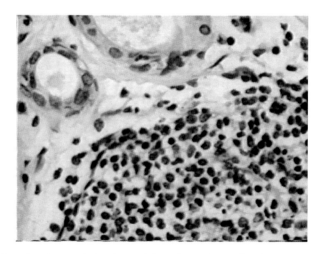

Plate 17 (See also Fig. 45.2) Histology of the minor salivary gland.

Table 24.1 NICE/BSR guidelines for anti-TNF therapy TA130

Time	DAS
Start	>5.1
6 months	Falls by 1.2 or is <3.2
Subsequently	>1.2 below initial level

Source: NICE Technology Appraisal TA130 (http://guidance.nice.org.uk/TA130).

Further reading

Funovits J, Aletaha D, Bykerk V, *et al.* (2010). The 2010 American College of Rheumatology/
European League Against Rheumatism classification criteria for rheumatoid arthritis:
methodological report phase I. *Ann Rheum Dis*; **69**: 1589–95.

Luqmani R, Hennell S, Estrach C, *et al.* (2009). British Society for Rheumatology and British
Health Professionals in Rheumatology guideline for the management of rheumatoid
arthritis (after the first 2 years). *Rheumatology*; **48**: 436–9.

Case 25

Part 1

A 72-year-old Caucasian female presented with rapid-onset, painful, and disabling dactylitis of both second toes (Fig. 25.1). She had a past history of mechanical low back pain. Since the development of dactylitis she suffered general malaise, pain all over, and night sweats. On examination she was distressed and anxious, afebrile, and nor-motensive, with widespread hyperalgesia but no significant abnormality apart from dactylitis of both second toes. In particular, there were no skin, hair, or nail lesions. During the following few months the dactylitis migrated between different toes, but was always present in at least two toes. The pain, fever, and malaise troubled her to such an extent that she became depressed. She was treated with paracetamol, NSAIDs, amitriptyline, and morphine sulphate, all of which were ineffective. Intravenous methylprednisolone had a transient effect on the inflammatory response. DMARDs (methotrexate, leflunomide, and sulfasalazine) were also ineffective.

Investigations showed the following:

- Hb 12.7 g/dL initially   10.1 g/dL after 4 months (MCV 88 fL)
- Platelets 430 × 10⁹/L initially   856 × 10⁹/L after 4 months
- CRP 80 mg/L initially   160 mg/L after 4 months
- WCC 14.5 × 10⁹/L initially   22.1 × 10⁹/L after 4 months
- Lymphocytes 7.2 × 10⁹/L initially   11.7 × 10⁹/L after 4 months
- Urinalysis was unremarkable throughout.

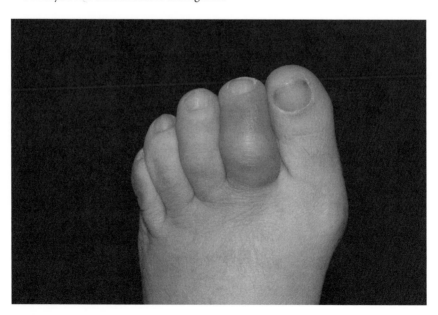

Fig. 25.1 (See also Plate 12) Dactylitis of left second toe.

Questions—Part 1

1. What is the differential diagnosis for dactylitis?
2. What other investigations would you undertake in this case?

Answers

1. What is the differential diagnosis for dactylitis?

Dactylitis is the inflammation of a finger or toe, affecting any of the structures within a digit. There are many causes, the most common of which is an association with inflammatory arthritis, sarcoidosis, or sickle cell disease. With increasing globalization, infection-related dactylitis associated with tuberculosis and congenital syphilis should be considered. Blistering dactylitis associated with group A β-haemolytic streptococci or *Staphylococcus aureus* infection is a rare complication of these ubiquitous infections.

- Dactylitis associated with inflammatory arthritis, particularly seronegative spondyloarthritis, is a diffuse painful swelling of a digit caused by a combination of flexor tenosynovitis, soft tissue oedema, synovitis, enthesitis, and bone oedema. It is most commonly seen in psoriatic arthritis (up to one-third of patients), but also occurs with all seronegative spondyloarthritides and reactive arthritis. Often dactylitis manifests as 'sausage-like' digits and involves a few fingers or toes asymmetrically. Clinical examination is usually sufficient for diagnosis, but in severe cases the dactylitis may resemble cellulitis or osteomyelitis. Most cases are self-limiting and DMARD treatment is reserved for persistent cases or those with associated arthritis.

- Sarcoid dactylitis is a rare manifestation of sarcoidosis, occurring in about 0.2% of patients, and is often associated with lupus pernio. Non-caseating granulomas invade the bones and adjacent soft tissue, leading to fusiform swellings which are usually bilateral, asymmetrical, and painless. Serum angiotensin-converting enzyme (ACE) level may be raised and there may be associated hypercalcaemia and hilar lymphadenopathy. Diagnosis is confirmed by tissue biopsy from the digit or other skin lesions.

- Sickle cell disease dactylitis is caused by infarction of bone marrow during painful vaso-occlusive crises. It most commonly occurs during early childhood and is sometimes the first manifestation of the disease. Clinically, it is characterized by sudden onset of a warm tender global swelling of the hands or feet, often with fever and leucocytosis. X-ray appearance may resemble that of osteomyelitis, with a 'moth-eaten' periostitis and focal osteosclerosis. Haemoglobin electrophoresis is used to test for sickle cell disease.

- Tuberculous dactylitis is a rare extrapulmonary manifestation of tuberculosis caused by osteomyelitis extending into digit soft tissue. It usually presents as a painful soft tissue swelling around the diaphysis of the involved bone. An abnormal CXR points towards the diagnosis, which may need to be confirmed by tissue biopsy.

- Syphilitic dactylitis is a manifestation of congenital syphilis resulting from transplacental transmission of *Treponema pallidum*. The spirochetes invade perichondrium, periosteum, cartilage, bone marrow, and sites of active endochondral ossification. The dactylitis is bilateral and symmetric. Syphilis is confirmed by screening tests for syphilis (IgM/IgG combined enzyme immunoassay (EIA), VDRL, or *Treponema pallidum* haemagglutination (TPHA) tests).

♦ Blistering distal dactylitis is an infection of the anterior fat pad of the volar surface of the distal part of the finger or toe, most often caused by group A β-haemolytic streptococci and occasionally staphylococcus aureus. It characteristically manifests as a tense bulla which covers the anterior fat pad, proximal and lateral nail folds. Usually there are no constitutional symptoms, and treatment is with excision, drainage. Systemic antibiotics are usually given to prevent spread of the infection.

2. What other investigations would you undertake in this case?

This woman's painful dactylitis in association with systemic symptoms and raised inflammatory markers meant that investigations were needed to exclude an underlying seronegative inflammatory arthritis, connective tissue disease, vasculitis, and the infectious causes of dactylitis. The level of constitutional upset and inflammatory response, which was disproportionate to the clinical signs, prompted a search for occult malignancy.

Further normal tests were:

♦ liver function, renal function, serum calcium, bone biochemistry

♦ ANA, ANCA, rheumatoid factor

♦ serum ACE, QuantiFERON® test for tuberculosis

♦ immunoglobulin, electrophoresis, and urine for Bence-Jones proteins

♦ infection screen—blood, urine, throat culture

♦ echocardiogram.

Imaging was as follows:

♦ MRI spine to look for spinal infection, metastatic disease, and infection.

Screening for occult malignancy involved:

♦ CT of chest, abdomen and pelvis

♦ upper and lower GI endoscopy

♦ breast screening

♦ pelvic ultrasound.

All investigations in this patient were normal except for the blood film which showed a persistent lymphocytosis. Peripheral blood leucocyte immunophenotyping revealed a neoplastic B-cell clone, consistent with a diagnosis of chronic lymphocytic leukaemia (CLL). A diagnosis of paraneoplastic syndrome was proposed. She was treated with chlorambucil and her dactylitis symptoms and inflammatory response settled as her white cell count normalized.

Questions—Part 2

3. What are the rheumatological manifestations of paraneoplastic syndromes?

4. How should a patient with suspected paraneoplastic arthritis be managed?

5. What is the prognosis of a patient with paraneoplastic arthritis?

Answers

3. What are the rheumatological manifestations of paraneoplastic syndromes?

Malignant disease can affect the musculoskeletal system by direct invasion, metastasis, synovial reaction to juxta-articular masses, and indirectly by the effects of a distant tumour. A wide variety of paraneoplastic syndromes can occur involving multiple organ systems, including the musculoskeletal system.

The paraneoplastic syndromes are thought to be caused by a humoral response to a malignancy, and can be defined by the following criteria:

◆ They occur during the course of an identified malignant disease or precede clinical evidence of a malignancy.

◆ Symptoms cannot be the result of direct tumour invasion or compression.

◆ Symptoms improve with treatment of the underlying neoplasm.

Presentation is often atypical with a rapid onset, and symptoms and signs may be migratory. The systemic inflammatory response may be disproportionate to the arthritis as in this patient's case. Autoantibody screening tests are usually negative, and response to corticosteroids and immunosuppressive agents is poor.

Inflammatory myopathies, seronegative rheumatoid arthritis, and some atypical vasculitides are the most frequently reported paraneoplastic rheumatological diseases, although paraneoplastic scleroderma-like and lupus-like syndromes, erythema nodosum, and Raynaud's syndrome have also been described.

Adult patients presenting with inflammatory myositis (dermatomyositis and polymyositis) have a significant malignancy association. Patients presenting with PMR symptoms who are younger than age 50 with an ESR <40 or >100, and who respond poorly to corticosteroids, should be considered for age-appropriate malignancy screening.

4. How should a patient with suspected paraneoplastic arthritis be managed?

Paraneoplastic arthritis is not common but it often presents before the malignancy itself, on average by 3 months. Therefore it is important to undertake age-specific screening for malignancy in anyone in whom it is suspected. Treatment of the malignancy often leads to a resolution of the rheumatological disease. In one case series, 12 out of the 13 patients with paraneoplastic arthritis had resolution of their joint symptoms with chemotherapy or tumour resection. The mean age of initial presentation was 58 years (range 28–85 years). Sixty per cent of paraneoplastic arthritis is caused by adenocarcinoma of the lung; therefore it is important to have a higher index of suspicion with smokers. Although both solid and haematological malignancies can cause paraneoplastic arthritis, it is more common with solid malignancies. There is no relation between the type of arthritis and the underlying tumour type.

3. What is the prognosis of a patient with paraneoplastic arthritis?

The prognosis is linked to the progression of the malignancy. With a high index of suspicion, malignancies occurring as part of paraneoplastic arthritis tend to be detected at an earlier stage than usual. Therefore the chances of survival are often higher for patients with paraneoplastic arthritis than for those without.

In this case a recurrence of the patient's lymphocytosis was heralded by a recurrence of the dactylitis. It is important to be aware of this, as rheumatological symptoms can serve as an early warning for tumour recurrence, with early detection leading to an improved treatment outcome. However, not all cases of tumour relapse involve a recurrence of the rheumatological symptoms.

Further reading

Racanelli V, Marcella P, Minoia C, Favoino E, Perosa F (2008). Rheumatic disorders as paraneoplastic syndromes *Autoimmun Rev*; **7**: 352–8.

Morel J, Deschamps V, Toussirot E, *et al.* (2008). Characteristics and survival of 26 patients with paraneoplastic arthritis. *Ann Rheum Dis*; **67**: 244–7.

Olivieri E, Scarano A, Padula V (2006). Dactylitis: a term for different digit diseases. *Scand J Rheumatol*; **35**: 333–40.

Case 26

A 40-year-old male presented with a 3-week history of multiple transient focal neurological events. On the first occasion, he woke up with left-sided weakness and incoherent speech lasting for a few minutes. This was followed within a few days by episodes of right hemiparesis and expressive dysphasia lasting up to 30 minutes. These symptoms were associated with a constant occipital headache, worse towards the end of day, which was helped with analgesia. He had no relevant past medical history and had never smoked. On examination, his blood pressure was 135/85 mmHg. He had minimal ataxia on heel–toe walking, but his neurological examination was otherwise normal.

Investigations showed the following:

- Normal haematological and biochemical studies
- Normal inflammatory markers
- Negative ANA, ANCA, RF, cryoglobulins, normal complement
- Negative thrombophilia screen
- Normal CXR
- ECG: normal sinus rhythm
- Normal transthoracic echocardiogram
- MRI and MRA of the brain are shown in Figs 26.1 and 26.2
- CSF: opening pressure 8 cmH$_2$O, glucose 3.8 mmol/L (blood 5.8 mmol/L), protein 477 mg/L, lymphocytes 20/mm^3, no red cells, and no oligoclonal bands.

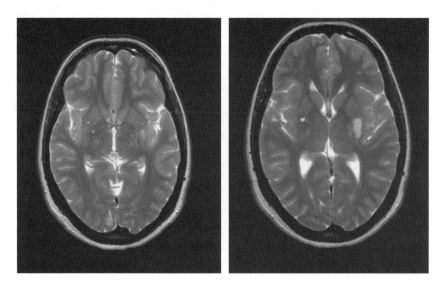

Fig. 26.1 T$_2$-weighted MR images of the brain with gadolinium.

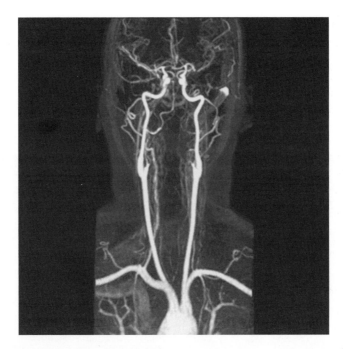

Fig. 26.2 Magnetic resonance angiogram.

Questions

1. What does the MRI and MRA brain (Figs 26.1 and 26.2) show?
2. What is the differential diagnosis?
3. What other investigations should be considered?
4. How would you treat this condition?

Answers

1. What does the MRI and MRA brain (Figs 26.1 and 26.2) show?

The MR images with gadolinium demonstrate small focal enhancing parenchymal lesions (Fig. 26.3, arrows). There were multiple lesions of varying ages in the left posterior putamen, internal capsule, and right basal ganglia. The MRA shows reduced calibre of the left middle cerebral artery (Fig. 26.4, arrow).

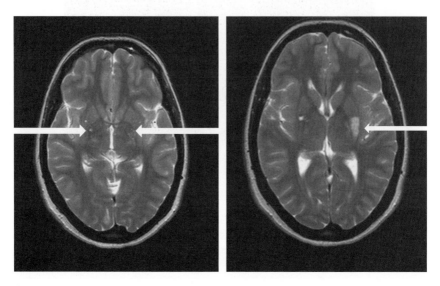

Fig. 26.3 T$_2$-weighted MR images of brain with gadolinium demonstrating small focal enhancing parenchymal lesions (arrows).

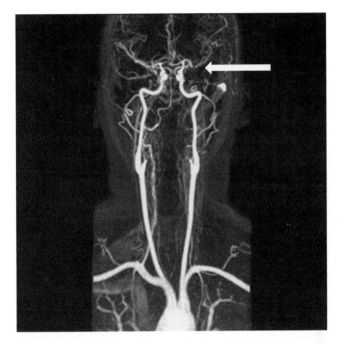

Fig. 26.4 MRA angiogram showing reduced calibre of left middle cerebral artery (arrow).

2. What is the differential diagnosis?

This patient has vascular disease affecting a number of vessels of varying calibre and causing lesions of different ages. The differential diagnoses are:

◆ primary angiitis of the CNS (PACNS)

◆ reversible cerebral vasoconstrictive syndromes (RCVSs)

◆ secondary CNS vasculitis.

Secondary forms of CNS vasculitis may occur in many conditions including the following:

◆ Infections: HIV, varicella zoster virus (VZV), hepatitis C, syphilis.

◆ Drugs: amphetamines, cocaine, heroin, ephedrine, phenylpropanolamine.

◆ Lymphoproliferative disease: Hodgkin's and non-Hodgkin's lymphoma.

◆ Systemic vasculitis: PAN, MPA, BD, WG, CSS.

◆ Connective tissue diseases: SLE, Sjögren's syndrome.

◆ Other: radiation, graft versus host disease.

Infections of the CNS with HIV, VZV, hepatitis C, and syphilis may result in a similar clinical picture to that of primary CNS vasculitis. VZV cerebral angiitis generally affects older patients and may be preceded by a clinical zoster infection. Diagnosis is confirmed by a positive VZV IgM in the CSF. HIV may be the primary infection causing a CNS vasculitis or associated with an opportunistic infection such as neurosyphilis. Hepatitis C may cause a CNS vasculitis without cryoglobuli-naemia. Other infections causing a CNS vasculitis are *Borrelia burgdorferi*, *Bartonella*, *Mycobacterium tuberculosis*, and cysticercosis.

Most systemic vasculitides may involve the CNS, but the most commonly report-ed are PAN, BD, and the ANCA-associated vasculitides.

Results of investigations so far did not support a diagnosis of systemic inflamma-tory disease, lymphoproliferative disorder, APS, infection, metabolic disorder, or a thromboembolic disease.

RCVSs are an important differential and may present with similar clinical and radiological features to CNS vasculitis. Young female patients characteristically present with a severe acute ('thunderclap') headache with or without neurological signs but without evidence of a subarachnoid haemorrhage. CSF analysis is usually normal. Multifocal segmental cerebral artery vasoconstriction is best demonstrated on angiography showing multiple vessel involvement in multiple beds, and the changes are reversible within 12 weeks. It is twice as common in females, and tends to occur in the 20–40-year-old age group. MRI scans may be normal but can show infarction resulting from hypoperfusion and small subarachnoid haemorrhages resulting from reperfusion. It is a self-resolving condition, but may be treated with calcium-channel blockers and occasionally high-dose steroids. It is less likely in this case where the disease onset is insidious and the CSF is abnormal.

PACNS is a rare form of vasculitis and is of unknown cause. Evidence of systemic inflammation is characteristically absent. Presentation can be extremely variable but generally includes multifocal neurological signs and symptoms with headache or altered mental states. Diagnostic criteria for PACNS were proposed by Calabrese and Malleck in 1998, and include all of the following:

- An acquired neurological deficit that remains unexplained after thorough evaluation.

- Either high-probability angiographic evidence or histopathologic demonstration of angiitis within the CNS.

- No evidence of systemic vasculitis or any other condition to which the angiographic or pathological condition could be attributed.

Clinical subsets of PACNS comprise granulomatous angiitis of the CNS (GACNS), which accounts for 20% of cases, spinal cord and mass lesion presentations, and atypical cases where granulomatous angiitis is associated with GCA, sarcoidosis, and amyloidosis.

GACNS is more common in males with a male-to-female ratio of 3:2 and a median age of 50 years. It has a variable onset and is often associated with a 3–6-month pro-dromal illness. The major symptoms include headache, strokes, or encephalopathy, but presentation may include recurrent transient ischaemic attacks, seizures, cognitive or behavioural changes, myelopathy, and ataxia. The CSF is abnormal in 80–90% of patients with PACNS with mild to moderate leucocytosis and elevated protein.

This case was most likely to be a presentation of PACNS in view of the multiple focal neurological events with headache, the CSF findings, demonstration of multiple vessel involvement on MRI, and absence of any other abnormal investigations.

3. What other investigations should be considered?

A brain and leptomeningeal biopsy is the gold standard investigation for the diagnosis of PACNS. The histological features consist of granulomatous inflammation, fibrinoid necrosis of vessel walls, or lymphocytic infiltrates. Sensitivity may be low due to skip lesions and sampling error but can be improved by using MRI to select enhancing lesions.

Further imaging studies include formal cerebral angiography, computed tomography angiography, and 18-fluorodeoxyglucose positron emission tomography. Cerebral angiography can demonstrate disease of larger and medium-sized vessels (e.g. stenosis and aneurysms), but it is less sensitive for disease in smaller vessels although it has higher resolution than MRA.

Angiography may be normal in 40% of cases where the diseased vessel is small and is termed high probability in 40% of cases where vessels show definite involvement.

Serum and CSF studies should be performed to detect viral, bacterial, and atypical infections.

4. How would you treat this condition?

There have been no randomized controlled trials of the treatment of CNS vasculitis, and management is based on extrapolation of protocols for other systemic vasculitides with severe organ involvement. This patient should be managed in collaboration with a neurologist. Current practice is to use pulse cyclophosphamide and glucocorticoid regimens to achieve remission followed by azathioprine, methotrexate, or mycophenolate mofetil for maintenance. Adjuvant treatment includes prevention of opportunistic infection and osteoporosis.

This patient responded well to a course of pulsed cyclophosphamide and oral corticosteroids, with resolution of symptoms and return to normal function. He started maintenance treatment with mycophenolate mofetil and has been carefully followed up as the relapse rate of the condition is estimated at 25%. Early recognition of disease and prompt treatment is likely to improve outcome.

Further reading

Birnbaum J, Hellmann DB (2009). Primary angiitis of the CNS. *Arch Neurol*; **66**: 704–9.

Calabrese LH, Malleck JA (1988). Primary angiitis of the central nervous system. *Medicine*; **67**: 20–39.

Calabrese LH (2007). Narrative review: reversible cerebral vasoconstriction syndromes. *Ann Int Med*; **146**: 34–44.

Calabrese LH, Duna GF (2008). Vasculitis of the central nervous system. In: Ball E, Bridges SL (eds) *Vasculitis* (2nd edn). Oxford: Oxford University Press.

Hajj-Ali RA, Calabrese LH (2009). Central nervous system vasculitis. *Curr Opin Rheumatol*; **21**: 10–18.

Küker W (2007). Cerebral vasculitis: imaging signs revisited. *Neuroradiology*; **49**: 471–9.

Case 27

A 26-year-old woman, who had been working part-time as a waitress and training to be a beauty therapist, was referred to the rheumatology outpatient department with severe pain and weakness in her legs. The patient stated that her leg symptoms occurred as a result of a fall at her workplace 6 months previously when she slipped on wet tiles in the restaurant. There was initial bruising of her left calf and thigh. Her employers were not sympathetic, denying that the floor was wet. She was in the process of taking legal action against them. She had not been able to work since because her legs were too painful; her mobility was severely affected and she was confined to her home. Her parents were present during the consultation and they provided the history. The patient was tearful and did not say very much, but complained of fatigue and pain. There was no past medical history apart from migraines and dysmenorrhea.

On examination the patient was noted to be overweight. She could not walk without her father assisting her. Both legs had normal tone; there was a global weakness of her legs related to pain. The skin was cool, especially below her knees, and she described marked hyperalgesia of the skin from the mid-thigh downwards. Reflexes were normal and the joints were normal apart from exquisite pain on movement.

Questions

1. What is the diagnosis?
2. Would the presence of more widespread trigger points and sleep disturbance change the diagnosis?
3. What is the approach to management?
4. What is the role of pharmacotherapy for neuropathic pain?
5. What are the risk factors for this patient having a poor outcome?

Answers

1. What is the diagnosis?

The working diagnosis is that of a complex regional pain syndrome (CRPS). This condition encompasses a diversity of painful conditions, often following trauma, coupled with abnormal regulation of blood flow and sweating, trophic changes, and oedema of the skin. The excruciating pain and autonomic dysfunction is disproportionate to any inciting event. CRPS type I is formally identified as reflex sympathetic dystrophy. CRPS type II is the term that describes the condition when it coexists with documented nerve injury.

CRPS I may follow trivial injury. Clinical features include allodynia, hyperalgesia, oedema, pseudo-motor and vasomotor abnormalities, and subsequent trophic changes. This results in a diminution in quality of life and overall reduction in health. There is an interplay with the organic features of the reflex sympathetic dystrophy and the non-organic pain modulation disorder. A physical trauma is often the precipitating event and becomes a point of fixation, particularly when there is a legal claim or compensation is sought.

2. Would the presence of more widespread trigger points and sleep disturbance change the diagnosis?

The presence of widespread trigger points and sleep disturbance with fatigue would raise the possibility that the patient had developed fibromyalgia. The definition encompasses pain and tenderness that affects muscles and tendons over the whole body and continues for more than 3 months. It is called a 'syndrome' because it is a collection of symptoms, rather than a disease. It is almost always present in association with non-restorative sleep. There is evidence that in these patients' psychological conditions, including depression, panic disorders, anxiety, and post-traumatic stress, may play a part. Genetic factors may also play a role in the pathogenesis of a fibromyalgia syndrome. Personality factors may also be involved. Buskila and colleagues have analysed coping styles of fibromyalgia patients with specific emphasis on the differences between those patients with and without post-traumatic stress. The psychological concept of 'suppression' as a coping style is significantly more common in fibromyalgia patients with comorbid post-traumatic stress.

3. What is the approach to management?

Management of CRPS I requires a clear therapeutic plan which needs the full participation and cooperation of the patient and family. Understanding the process and its presentation is paramount to the success of treatment. The physiotherapist often leads in the management. A graded exercise programme, training the patient to use their legs fully, should be commenced as soon as possible. Altering sensory stimuli such as hot, cold, light touch, and vibration are helpful in re-training nerves. Balance and proprioception are often lost early and need to be worked on. There is some evidence that mirror therapy may be helpful in CRPS I.

The primary tool of mirror therapy is a mirror from which the patient receives visual feedback in order to 'train' the brain to configure a new 'body map'. This so-called map is the mental representation that allows a person to be aware of where each component of the body is at all times, even in complete darkness. The feedback that is gained from the normal limb is used to train the painful limb.

Clinical psychology and pain-management strategies need to proceed alongside the physical therapies. The losses to self-esteem, work, and health need to be addressed, and their meaning to the patient needs to be explored. Acupuncture and transcutaneous electrical nerve stimulation (TENS) may have some value in the relief of pain, but the evidence base for these treatments is poor.

4. What is the role of pharmacotherapy for neuropathic pain?

Pharmacotherapy has a role in the management of neuropathic pain. Drugs such as tricyclic antidepressants and serotonin reuptake inhibitors may be useful. Noradrenaline and serotonin are important mediators of descending inhibition of noxious signalling and are important in stress response pathways. Meta-analyses have demonstrated the efficacy of tricyclic antidepressants in fibromyalgia. Selective serotonin reuptake inhibitors have limited efficacy. Anticonvulsants such as gabapentin and pregabalin, which affect calcium flux and the release of excitatory amino acids, have been shown to be useful. The analgesic tramadol, which is a μ-opioid receptor agonist inhibiting noradrenaline and serotonin reuptake, has been shown to be useful.

There has been some role for the use of bisphosphonates and also regional nerve blocks, in particular guanethidine.

5. What are the risk factors for this patient having a poor outcome?

There are a number of predisposing factors for the development of a more widespread pain disorder in this patient. She had had a work-related injury, was taking legal action, was currently not working, had put on weight, and had lost self-esteem and independence. There is a suggestion that there may be an unhealthy enmeshment with her family. The ongoing compensation claim will, in itself, increase anxiety. She will need to undergo numerous assessments by independent expert witnesses, and it is likely that she will be required to be assessed by a psychiatrist. She may undergo covert video surveillance by legal teams, which can be very stressful. Furthermore, if she feels that she will achieve a significant financial gain from the compensation, there may be a 'secondary gain' in her not responding to treatment. Her lack of self-esteem and weight gain may diminish her interest in her beauty therapy course and amplify her isolation and low mood. If she becomes secondarily depressed and sedated by medication, her volition levels will be low. With prolonged reduction in physical activity, her aerobic fitness, proprioception, and muscle tone will all be reduced, making it more difficult to rehabilitate.

Further reading

Ablin JN, Cohen H, Neumann L, Caplan Z, Buskila D (2008). Coping styles in fibromyalgia: effective co-morbid posttraumatic stress disorder. *Rheumatol Int*; **28**: 649–56.

Case 28

A 26-year-old woman was referred by her GP with an 8-year history of Raynaud's syndrome. She described several occasions where she had had infected ischaemic ulcers on her feet. She smoked 15 cigarettes a day and was on the combined oral contraceptive pill. She was seen by the registrar, who noted spindled fingers with distal pulp atrophy. Her fingers and toes were cold and had a dusky blue discoloration. Investigations were arranged and she was advised to stop smoking. Her ENA was positive for anticentromere antibody. Lung function tests showed a reduced TLCO of 72%. The chest CT scan was normal, as was an echocardiogram.

Questions

1. What is the diagnosis?
2. What does the positive anticentromere antibody mean?
3. Why is smoking cessation especially important in this patient?
4. Why was an echocardiogram arranged and how will this influence treatment?
5. What treatment approaches are there for Raynaud's syndrome?

Answers

1. What is the diagnosis?

The diagnosis is limited cutaneous systemic sclerosis. This is a subset of scleroderma which is characterized by the CREST syndrome: **C**alcinosis, **R**aynaud's syndrome, o**E**sphageal involvement **S**clerodactyly, and **T**elangiectasia. The calcinosis most frequently occurs in areas of relative ischaemia such as the fingers and the tips of the ears. The cold dusky fingers suggest Raynaud's syndrome, and distal pulp atrophy with spindled fingers is consistent with sclerodactyly. Oesophageal dysmotility may cause chronic reflux with dyspepsia; a barium swallow would help to elucidate this. Telangiectasia is often seen on the fingers and face as well as on the upper chest. This form of scleroderma contrasts with the diffuse cutaneous systemic sclerosis where there is more widespread skin thickening and major organ involvement such as parenchymal lung and renal disease.

2. What does positive anticentromere antibody mean?

The presence of a positive anticentromere antibody (usually IgG) is associated with the CREST syndrome. In a study from the Mayo Clinic, serum samples from 539 subjects with scleroderma were screened for the presence of the antibody and it was found in 11%, most of whom had features of the CREST syndrome either independently or in association with primary biliary cirrhosis. The antibody was rarely found in patients with rapidly advancing or diffuse scleroderma. The anticentromere antibody is a useful indicator in patients with early scleroderma as it may help to predict what pattern of scleroderma will evolve. Furthermore, it is associated with the development of pulmonary hypertension.

3. Why is smoking cessation especially important in this patient?

Smoking cessation is important as smoking exacerbates Raynaud's syndrome. There is evidence that smoking sensitizes the peripheral vasculature to the vasoconstricting effects. This is in part due to sensitization mediated by the inhibition of endothelial prostacyclin synthesis. The reduction in this patient's gas transfer suggests that she has already developed intrinsic lung disease secondary to smoking, and this would be further supported by a reduction in the FEV_1/FVC ratio. Smoking will also increase her risk of developing cardiovascular disease.

4. Why was an echocardiogram arranged and how will this influence treatment?

The echocardiogram was arranged to assess pulmonary vessel hypertension. Patients with CREST syndrome and anticentromere antibodies may have associated pulmonary artery hypertension, an important cause of mortality. These symptoms may initially be non-specific or silent, and consequently pulmonary hypertension is often under-recognized until the late stages. Early treatment is associated with a better outcome. Echocardiography is a useful pointer, but right-heart catheterization remains the gold standard. Conventional treatments for pulmonary hypertension are based on non-endothelial-specific drugs such as warfarin, oxygen, and diuretics. Calcium-channel blockers are often ineffective. Intravenous or aerosol-inhaled prostacyclin has been used and is the first-line treatment for the most severe cases. Phosphodiesterase-5 inhibitors (e.g. sildenafil) have been shown to be useful. Endothelin-1 is a potent vasoconstrictor and smooth muscle mitogen. The orally administered dual endothelin-receptor antagonist bosentan has been shown to improve exercise capacity and cardiopulmonary haemodynamics in patients with pulmonary arterial hypertension. However, administration is limited by cost.

5. What treatment approaches are there for Raynaud's syndrome?

Raynaud's syndrome is episodic vasospasm of peripheral arteries resulting in pallor followed by cyanosis and then redness due to hyperperfusion. There is associated pain and sometimes paraesthesia, and occasionally ulceration of the fingers, toes, pinnae of the ears, and tip of the nose may occur. Treatment should initially be conservative and non-pharmacological. Patients should be advised to increase their core body temperature by dressing warmly and using thermal underwear and heated gloves. Avoiding the cold and smoking cessation are important. Calcium-channel antagonists such as nifedipine may be helpful, but are often limited in their use by side effects such as hypotension, peripheral oedema, and headaches. Other drugs such as angiotenson II inhibitors, selective serotonin reuptake inhibitors, and the phosphodiesterase-5 inhibitors may be useful, but may also be limited by side effects. Topical nitrates can cause headaches and flushing. Intermittent prostacyclin infusions may be useful and are often given at the start of the cold season. Their effect rarely lasts longer than 8–10 weeks.

Further reading

Carroll WD, Dhillon R (2003). Sildenafil as a treatment for pulmonary hypertension. *Arch Dis Child*; **88**: 827–8.

McHugh NJ, Csuka M, Watson H, *et al.* (1988). Infusion of iloprost, a prostacyclin analogue, for treatment of Raynaud's phenomenon in systemic sclerosis. *Ann Rheum Dis*; **47**: 43–7.

Powell FC, Winkelmann RK, Venencie-Lemarchand F (1984). The anticentromere antibody: disease specificity and clinical significance. *Mayo Clin Proc*; **59**: 700–6.

Rubin LJ, Badesch DB, Barst RJ, *et al.* (2002). Bosentan therapy for pulmonary arterial hypertension. *N Engl J Med*; **346**: 896–903.

Case 29

A 36-year-old previously fit green-keeper at a golf course was admitted to the infectious diseases unit with a 5-week history of puffy hands, weakness of the arms and legs, and fatigue. He was finding it difficult to stand from sitting and had episodes of night-time fever. There was no travel history. He owned a dog. There was no history of tick bites, no contact with other individuals with a similar history, no past medical history, and no relevant family history. He had been a smoker of 15 cigarettes a day since age 19 years. Specific enquiry excluded Raynaud's syndrome, dryness of eyes or mouth, rashes, or difficulty in swallowing and there was no change in bowel habit.

Examination revealed oedema of hands with scaly patches over the knuckles, pitting oedema of the feet up to the knees, and purple scaling over the eyelids. His temperature was 37°C, pulse 104 beats/min, and BP 120/65 mmHg. His chest was clinically clear and cardiac examination was normal. His muscle power was reduced to four-fifths in a proximal distribution. Reflexes were normal. Tone was difficult to assess as there appeared to be oedema of the muscles. There was a suggestion of synovitis at the wrists.

Questions

1. Which diseases will the infectious disease physicians want to exclude before referring the patient to rheumatology?
2. Which routine blood investigations would be helpful in the context of proximal muscle weakness and joint inflammation?
3. Which radiological investigations would be helpful in making a diagnosis?
4. How do the immunological blood tests help with the diagnosis and management?
5. What is the treatment for this patient with inflammatory muscle disease?
6. What are the other organ systems that may become involved and how does this relate to the prognosis, compared with other inflammatory muscle diseases?

Answers

1. Which diseases will the infectious disease physicians want to exclude before referring the patient to rheumatology?

Viral infections such as adenovirus, Coxsackie virus (especially B4), influenza A and B, and HIV may all present with systemic inflammation and features of a myositis. Bacterial infections are less likely, but those that affect muscle include staphylococci and streptococci, *Borrelia burgdorferi*, *Mycobacterium*, and *Mycoplasma*. There may be elevated creatine phosphokinase (CPK) levels and non-specific myopathic changes including fibre necrosis and inflammatory infiltrate on biopsy. Parasitic infections are usually associated with an eosinophilia; these include *Toxoplasma*, *Trichinella*, microsporidia, *Echinococcus*, and *Schistosoma*.

2. Which routine blood investigations would be helpful in the context of proximal muscle weakness and joint inflammation?

The FBC may show mild anaemia of chronic disease and the platelet count may be elevated reflecting inflammation. Renal function should be checked since it can be affected by muscle inflammation and myoglobinuria. The ESR will be elevated in 50% of patients with inflammatory muscle disease, but commonly the CRP may not be increased to the same degree, as occurs in SLE and scleroderma. The muscle enzymes are often elevated: CPK is released from damaged muscle and is a helpful indicator of disease severity. Elevated CPK occurs in 90% when first seen. Increases occur with exacerbations and can precede the exacerbation by 5–6 weeks.

LDH, predominantly LDH-5, may increase without necessarily correlating with cardiac involvement. AST correlates with biopsy-proven muscle inflammation and is useful in combination with CPK. Aldolase may also be elevated.

The albumin should be checked to exclude hypoalbuminaemia and nephrotic syndrome in view of the peripheral oedema.

The results of the patient's blood tests were as follows:

- Hb 10.9 g/L; WBC 14.8×10^9/L; neutrophils 11.5×10^9/L
- Platelets 437×10^9/L
- ESR 112 mm/h; CRP 53 mg/L
- Creatinine 82 μmol/L; ALT 535 IU/L; ALP 141 IU/L; albumin 29 g/L; CPK 12231 IU/L
- Urine was a red–brown colour.

3. Which radiological investigations would be helpful in making a diagnosis?

A CXR is required for assessment of the lung fields and cardiac size The lungs may be involved in myositis because of diaphragmatic and intercostal muscle weakness.

This can result in ventilatory failure or aspiration. Interstitial lung disease is a particular feature of dermatomyositis associated with antisynthetase antibodies (such as the Jo-1 antibody). An acute interstitial pneumonitis leading to a fibrosing lung disease with poor prognosis occurs. A high-resolution CT (HRCT) scan of the lungs will be helpful in characterizing the lung disease. HRCT is also useful for assessing progression of pulmonary involvement and response to therapy. Pulmonary vasculitis and pulmonary hypertension may also occur.

Cardiac involvement is commonly asymptomatic but can contribute to mortality. ECG and echocardiography may demonstrate the major cardiac complications including conduction disturbances, arrhythmias, and myocarditis. Heart block occasionally requires pacing. The most common arrhythmias are extrasystoles and tachyarrhythmias. Pericardial effusions are seen in 5–25%, but are usually asymptomatic.

The muscles may be imaged using ultrasound or MRI scanning. MRI is increasingly used to detect inflammation or muscle damage and may also reflect response to treatment. MRI may be helpful in determining the optimal muscle to biopsy. Fatty infiltration and atrophy are seen best with T_1-weighted imaging and inflammation is seen best with T_2-weighted or STIR imaging. Gadolinium can also be used to highlight inflammation.

The patient's CXR was normal. Echocardiography showed a minimal pericardial effusion with normal systolic function. The muscle MRI showed widespread symmetrical myositis and significant subcutaneous oedema was also noted (Figs 29.1 and 29.2).

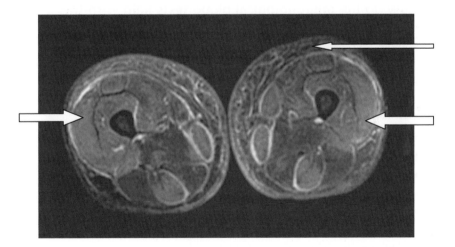

Fig. 29.1 Widespread symmetrical myositis affecting predominantly the quadriceps, (thick arrows) gracilis, and semitendinosis. There is also subcutaneous oedema (thin arrow).

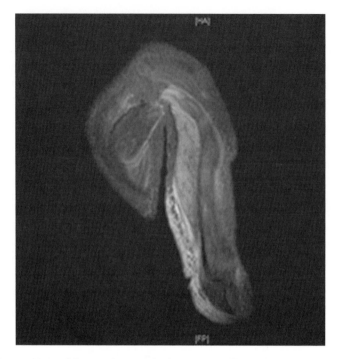

Fig. 29.2 Myositis involving predominantly the rotator cuff muscles, triceps, and coracobrachialis with subcutaneous oedema.

4. How do the immunological blood tests help with the diagnosis and management?

Inflammatory myopathies are considered to be autoimmune in nature. The antibodies in myositis may be myositis-specific antibodies (MSA) (Table 29.1) or myositis-associated antibodies (MAA). MAA are seen in patients with connective tissue diseases.

The patient's results were as follows:

◆ ANA negative
◆ Jo-1 positive
◆ ENA Ro positive
◆ RhF negative
◆ IgG 18.1 g/L; IgA 2.92 g/L; IgM 1.46 g/L.

This indicates a polyclonal rise in the immunoglobulins consistent with the acute phase response. The negative ANA is consistent with the absence of nuclear antibodies; both Jo-1 and Ro are cytosolic antibodies.

The anti-synthetase syndrome is that associated with Jo-1 or other aminoacyl tRNA synthetase antibodies. The clinical features are shown in Table 29.2. Twenty-five per cent of patients also have anti-Ro antibodies.

Table 29.1 Myositis-specific antibodies

	Anti-synthetase	Anti-SRP	Anti-Mi-2
Antigen	Anti-cytoplasmic Aminoacyl-tRNA synthetase Jo-1 histidyl-tRNA PL-7 threonyl-tRNA PL-12 alanyl-tRNA	Anti-cytoplasmic Signal recognition particle	Anti-nuclear Nuclear protein complex
Prevalence in PM/DM	20–50%	<5%	5–10%
Clinical association	Anti-synthetase syndrome	Severe resistant PM	Classic DM
HLA association	DRW52, DR3	DRW52, DR5	DRW53, DR7
Onset	Acute, spring	Very acute, winter	Acute
Clinical	PM » DM ILD (40–60%) Arthritis, deforming, but usually non-erosive Mechanic's hands Raynaud's syndrome	Severe PM Cardiac involvement	Classic DM Shawl sign rash Periungual erythema Cuticle overgrowth
Steroid response	Moderate	Poor	Good

DM, dermatomyositis; PM, polymyositis; ILD, interstitial lung disease.

Table 29.2 Features of the anti-synthetase syndrome

Clinical feature	Percentage (*n* = 47)
Myositis	100
Arthritis/arthralgia	94
Interstitial lung disease	89
Raynaud's syndrome	62
Fever	87
Mechanic's hands	71
DM rash	54
Anti-Ro antibody	25
Mortality	21
Female: male ratio	2.7

Adapted from Love LA *et al* (1991). *Medicine*; **70**: 360–74.

Muscle biopsy remains the gold standard test for muscle inflammation, although MRI is a useful non-invasive test and is helpful in monitoring the response to treatment. The biopsy in dermatomyositis shows perifascicular atrophy with shrinkage of muscle fibres at the edge of the fascicle. Inflammatory cells surround or invade the blood vessels. There is no invasion of normal muscle fibres as seen in polymyositis and inclusion body myositis.

5. What is the treatment of this patient with inflammatory muscle disease?

Treatment should be started without delay to avoid a poor outcome. Dermatomyositis and polymyositis respond to steroids; however, there is a lack of good-quality evidence. Treatment is usually with 1mg/kg prednisolone initially which is continued until the CPK has returned to normal and strength has improved (usually 4–6 weeks). Intravenous methylprednislone can be given for very ill patients. The response to treatment is often slower than is seen in SLE or rheumatoid arthritis, with a mean time to recovery of normal strength of around 3 months. The steroid dose is then gradually lowered. Steroid-sparing drugs such as methotrexate, azathioprine, mycophenolate mofetil, and leflunomide are increasingly being used. There is some evidence that in the anti-synthetase syndrome, patients are more likely to respond to methotrexate than to azathioprine. Other drugs that have shown benefit is small studies include ciclosporin and intravenous immunoglobulin.

The patient was commenced on prednislone 60 mg and methotrexate 15 mg/week.

6. What are the other organ systems that may become involved and how does this relate to the prognosis compared with other inflammatory muscle diseases?

Other organ involvement includes the lungs, heart, and skin. Lung function tests should be performed at base line and might show evidence of inflammatory lung disease.

The patient's lung function tests were as follows:

- ◆ PEFR   485 L/min   82% predicted
- ◆ VC   4.8 L   91% predicted
- ◆ FEV$_1$/VC   77%
- ◆ TLCO   11.53   96% predicted
- ◆ KCO   1.58   116% predicted

The lung function tests are essentially within the normal range. The HRCT, which was arranged because of the association of pulmonary involvement with the Jo-1 antibody, showed minimal lymphadenopathy and no interstitial lung involvement (Fig. 29.3). It would be reasonable to repeat this in cases where the patient developed symptoms, or if there is a change in lung function tests which should be performed annually.

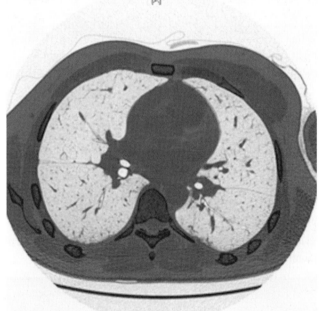

Fig. 29.3 HRCT of the chest—normal test.

Further reading

Joffe MM, Love LA, Leff RL, *et al.* (1993). Drug therapy of the idiopathic inflammatory myopathies:predictors of response to prednislone, azathioprine, and methotrexate and a comparison of their efficacy. *Am J Med*; **94**: 379–87.

Love LA, Leff RL, Fraser DD, *et al.* (1991). A new approach to the classification of inflammatory myopathy: myositis-specific autoantibodies define useful homogeneous patient groups. *Medicine*; **70**: 360–74.

Oddis CV (2008). Idiopathic inflammatory myopathies: treatment and assessment. In: Klippel J, Stone J, Crofford L, White P (eds) *Primer on the Rheumatic Diseases* (13th edn). New York: Springer; pp. 375–80.

Plotz PH, Dalakas M, Leff RL, Love LA, Miller FW, Cronin ME (1989). Current concepts in the idiopathic inflammatory myopathies: polymyositis, dermatomyositis and related disorders. *Ann Int Med*; **111**: 143–57.

Tomasova Studynkova J, Charvat F, Jarosova K, Venkovsky J (2007). The role of MRI in the assessment of polymyositis and dermatomyositis. *Rheumatology*; **46**: 1174–9.

Case 30

A 50-year-old Caucasian man presented with a 4-year history of fleeting large-joint arthritis affecting the knees and ankles. In the 6 months prior to presentation, he had developed night sweats, anorexia, diarrhoea, and associated weight loss. Examination revealed widespread lymphadenopathy, moderate hepatosplenomegaly, and a pyrexia of 38°C.

Investigations showed the following:

◆ Hb 8.4 g/L, MCV 72 fL

◆ RF and ACPA negative

◆ Anti-endomysial and tissue transglutaminase antibodies negative

◆ Immunoglobulins normal

◆ CRP 32 mg/L

◆ Blood cultures negative

◆ Upper and lower GI endoscopies were normal but there were numerous lymph nodes in the mesentery of the small bowel (Fig. 30.1).

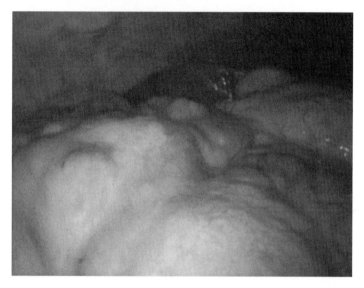

Fig. 30.1 (See also Plate 13) Mass of lymph nodes in the mesentery of the small bowel.

Questions—Part 1

1. What is the differential diagnosis in this case?

Answer

1. What is the differential diagnosis for this case?

The combination of constitutional upset, GI features, and arthritis raises a broad differential including infection, neoplasia, and IBD.

The most important differential to exclude is malignancy. The combination of widespread lymphadenopathy with hepatosplenomegaly, fever, and weight loss is most suggestive of lymphoma. An excision lymph node biopsy is needed to explore this diagnosis further. The picture of iron-deficiency anaemia also raises the possibility of GI malignancy, but the normal colonoscopy makes this less likely. Metastatic disease should also be considered, in particular from a primary prostate source in this case.

A detailed travel history is needed in order to focus screening for an underlying infectious cause. Common causes of lymphadenopathy include infectious mononucleosis, adenovirus, and CMV, but the prolonged history makes these somewhat unlikely. More chronic infectious causes to consider include giardiasis, amoebiasis, tuberculosis, brucellosis, histoplasmosis, and HIV.

IBD is a possible explanation for the diarrhoea and joint symptoms, but the normal macroscopic appearances on oesophagogastroduodenoscopy (OGD) and colonoscopy make this unlikely. BD can also give rise to diarrhoea with arthritis (see Case 39), but the absence of the characteristic oral and genital ulceration would be highly atypical. Similarly, musculoskeletal involvement has been reported in up to ~20% of patients with coeliac disease, but the negative anti-endomysial and tissue transglutaminase antibody results go against this diagnosis.

Other less likely possibilities include hyperthyroidism, malabsorption due to pancreatic disease, and other haematological diagnoses such as leukaemia.

Further investigations showed the following:

- HIV, CMV, and toxoplasma serology negative
- Tumour markers, including PSA, all negative
- Serum ACE negative
- CXR and TB ELISPOT negative
- Lymph node biopsy showed reactive changes only
- Bone marrow biopsy was normal apart from an increased number of eosinophils.

Questions—Part 2

2. What rare diagnosis can explain all of the above findings and how is the diagnosis made?

3. How would you manage this condition?

Answers

2. What rare diagnosis can explain all of the above findings and how is the diagnosis made?

Whipple's disease explains all of the above findings. Whipple's disease is due to an infection with *Tropheryma whippelii* and may cause diarrhoea, malabsorption and associated weight loss. Although the disease can occur worldwide, it commonly affects middle-aged Caucasian males. It is characterized by two phases: the prodromal stage with intermittent migratory arthralgia or arthritis, particularly affecting the knee, ankle, and wrist, and the steady state stage with typical manifestations including diarrhoea and weight loss. Other less common features include hepatosplenomegaly, ascites, myalgia, endocarditis, and neurological involvement.

Traditionally, periodic acid–Schiff (PAS) staining of a duodenal biopsy specimen has been the first-line diagnostic test (Fig. 30.2). The typical appearance is of foamy macrophages containing numerous PAS-positive organisms within the lamina propria. PAS-positive cells can be found in any affected organ. However, PAS staining is non-specific and can also be seen with other infectious agents including *Mycobacterium avium intracellulare*, *Corynebacterium*, and *Histoplasma*. Immunohistochemistry using *T. Whippelii*-specific antibodies improves histological specificity and sensitivity. In addition, a polymerase chain reaction (PCR)-based assay is now available in a few centres, but can be associated with false-positive detection in healthy individuals.

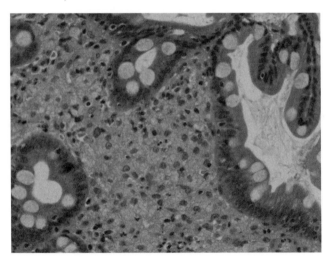

Fig. 30.2 (See also Plate 14) Photomicrographs of the duodenal biopsy showing macrophages containing PAS-positive granules.

3. How would you manage this condition?

Whipple's disease is potentially fatal if left untreated but responds to antibiotic therapy. Current recommendations for the treatment of Whipple's disease comprise induction therapy with intravenous antibiotics, commonly 14 days of ceftriaxone followed by continuation therapy with oral co-trimoxazole for 1–2 years. The response to treatment should be monitored closely as relapses are common, particularly in CNS disease which is associated with a high rate of recurrence after apparently successful treatment. In view of the risk of relapsing CNS disease, current recommendations favour co-trimoxazole over penicillins as it has blood–brain barrier penetration.

Further reading

Desnues B, Al Moussawi K, Fenollar F (2002). New insights into Whipple's disease and *Tropheryma whipplei* infections. *Microbes Infect*; **12**: 1102–10.

Puéchal X (2002). Whipple's disease. *Joint Bone Spine*; **69**: 133–40.

Case 31

A 28-year-old female runner presented with a 1-month history of right groin pain. She was a keen runner and ran competitively in marathons at a national level. Recently, she had increased her workload in preparation for a mountain challenge run. The pains were localized to her right groin and had come on insidiously but had gradually become worse over the preceding month. At presentation, she was complaining of pain in the right groin on walking and on any weight-bearing exercise. She denied any night pain. There was no history of an acute injury.

She had sustained a right navicular stress fracture in the past which was treated conservatively. She had been amenorrheic for 1 year and oligomenorrheic for 5 years prior to that. She limited her intake of energy rich foods. She changed her running shoes every 300–500 miles.

On examination her BMI was 17 kg/m². She had a limp due to pain on weight-bearing. There was no tenderness over the groin. Passive internal and external rotation of the hip exacerbated the pain only at the end range of movements. She had globally good muscle strength around the hip joint.

The DEXA scan showed *T*-scores of −2.6 at the spine and −2.8 at the hip.

The MRI of the hip joint is shown in Fig. 31.1.

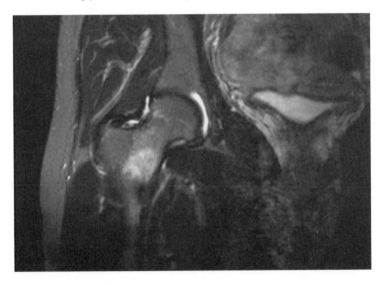

Fig. 31.1 MRI of the right hip.

Questions

1. What is the diagnosis?
2. What are the complications of this condition?
3. What other issues have been identified?
4. What other investigations would you request?
5. How would you treat this athlete?

Answers

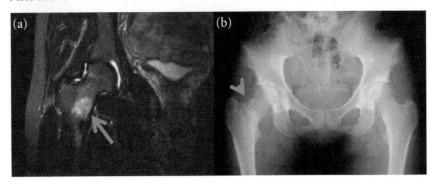

Fig. 31.2 (a) NOF stress fracture of the inferior surface on MRI (arrow). (b) NOF stress fracture of superior surface on X-ray (arrowhead).

1. What is the diagnosis?

The diagnosis is a stress fracture of the neck of the femur (NOF). Femoral neck stress fractures can be classified as superior surface or inferior surface (Fig. 31.2). In this case the stress fracture is on the inferior surface (Fig. 31.2). NOF stress fractures are more commonly seen on the inferior surface (80%) than on the superior surface (20%).

2. What are the complications of this condition?

NOF stress fractures are at high risk of progression to a complete displaced fracture with the possibility of avascular necrosis of the femoral head. Stress fractures of the superior surface are on the tension side of the femur; hence they are less stable and have a higher tendency to progress to a full fracture. Inferior surface fractures are on the compression side of the femur and are more stable.

3. What other issues have been identified?

This athlete is noted to have a disordered eating pattern and amenorrhea, and she is also osteoporotic. This triad of conditions is termed the 'female athlete triad'. The process is driven by an energy imbalance due to increased expenditure during exercise together with inadequate energy intake due to disordered eating patterns. This results in a low BMI and also shutting down of the hypothalamic–pituitary axis, resulting in menstrual disturbance. This in turn affects bone health and predisposes the athlete to stress fractures.

4. What other investigations would you request?

Further investigations should be carried out to investigate the metabolic bone issues and the amenorrhoea. Blood tests should include full blood count, bone profile, thyroid function, renal function, liver function, sex hormone profile, and vitamin D levels, and exclusion of malabsorption with endomysial or tissue transglutaminase antibodies. Prior to returning to sporting activities a formal biomechanical assessment should be considered, involving assessment of the athlete's walking and running biomechanics. This would involve gait analysis using motion detectors and high-speed cameras in a gait laboratory.

5. How would you treat this athlete?

There are two main issues that need to be addressed.

Treatment of the stress fracture

Treatment is either conservative or surgical. Conservative methods are favoured for NOF stress fractures of the inferior surface. Conservative treatment includes immediate non-weight-bearing rest with the use of crutches. The non-weight bearing period is usually guided by the patient's symptoms, but should last for at least 4–6 weeks. This is followed by a gradual introduction of activities, with a return to sport taking approximately 6 months. Surgical management is usually favoured for the treatment of NOF stress fractures of the superior surface.

Addressing the female athlete triad and associated issues

This is paramount to prevent further stress fractures. A multidisciplinary team approach with input from a sport and exercise medicine physician, a nutritionist, a psychologist and a coach is important. A considerable amount of time should be spent educating the athlete on the issues surrounding the female athlete triad and developing strategies to address these. The key would be to address the energy imbalance by increasing energy intake, optimizing training sessions, and ensuring adequate recovery time between training sessions. There could be some overlap with more serious eating disorders such as anorexia nervosa and bulimia. Hence, where appropriate, a psychiatrist may be added to the multidisciplinary team.

Further reading

Birch K (2005). Female athlete triad. In: Whyte G, Harries M, Williams C. *ABC of Sports and Exercise Medicine* (3rd edn). Oxford: Blackwell; pp. 50–3.
Brukner P, Khan K (2006). *Clinical Sports Medicine* (3rd edn). Sydney: McGraw-Hill.

Case 32

A 17-year-old male cricketer presented with a 2-month history of left-sided lower back pain. He was a right-arm fast bowler and had recently been selected to play for his county under-18 team. In addition, he played twice a week for his local club. Because of his county commitments, he had doubled the amount of overs he bowled per week. Bowling exacerbated the pain and rest relieved it. The back pain had become more intense since an episode 2 weeks previously when he had bowled at full speed and had developed excruciating lower back pain immediately afterwards.

On examination there was tenderness immediately to the left of the midline of the spine at the level of the L5 vertebrae. His gluteal and hamstring muscles had reduced flexibility. There was poor muscular control in the lumbar, pelvic, and hip regions, resulting in inadequate core stability during activities. Flexion of the spine was full and pain free, but extension exacerbated the pain. Passive rotation to the left while in lumbar spine extension caused significant discomfort. The MRI scan of the lumbar spine is shown in Fig. 32.1.

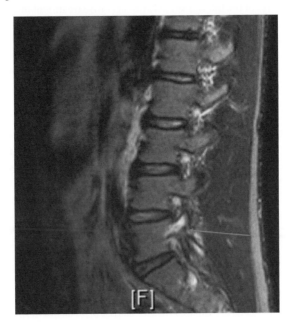

Fig. 32.1 MRI scan of the lumbar spine.

Questions

1. What does the MRI scan show?
2. Which sports predispose to this condition?
3. What factors have contributed to the development of this condition?
4. How would you manage this patient?
5. How would you prevent a recurrence of his problem?

Answers

1. What does the MRI scan show?

The MRI scan shows a stress fracture of the left pars interarticularis of the L5 vertebrae (see Fig. 32.1).

2. Which sports predispose to this condition?

Sports which involve repetitive extension and rotation of the spine predispose athletes to vertebral stress fracture. Examples include gymnastics, tennis, fast bowling in cricket, high jumping, pole vaulting, and weight-lifting.

3. What factors have contributed to the development of this condition?

There are intrinsic and extrinsic risk factors associated with a pars interarticularis stress fracture. Extrinsic factors include an increase in workload, for example in the current case an increase in the number of overs bowled per week. Changes in the playing surface or footwear may also contribute. Intrinsic factors include biomechanical errors in the bowling action. Bowling actions can be classified as one of three techniques: front on, side on, or a mixed technique where the lower half of the body is front on and the upper half is side on during delivery of the ball. It has been postulated that mixed bowling actions may increase the risk of developing pars interarticularis stress fractures. Other proposed intrinsic factors include poor core stability, gluteal and hamstring muscle inflexibility, and congenital defects of the neural arch of the vertebrae.

4. How would you manage this patient?

The patient should stop activities that exacerbate his pain. He should not resume extension activities, including bowling, until he can extend without any discomfort. A core stability strengthening programme should be initiated. Furthermore, inflexibility of the gluteal and hamstring muscles should be addressed via a stretching programme. The patient should be advised that it could take approximately 4 months to return to sport.

5. How would you prevent a recurrence of his problem?

The intrinsic and extrinsic factors that resulted in the injury must be addressed. A multidisciplinary team approach with good communication between the patient, his coach, and the physiotherapists is important. He may have to reduce either his club or his county commitments to reduce the number of overs bowled. The England and Wales Cricket Board has strict regulations regarding the maximum number of overs that any youth under the age of 19 can bowl per bowling spell and per day. Both he and his club should be advised to adhere to these regulations.

His bowling action should be assessed with his coach and he should continue his core stability strengthening programme and the hamstring and gluteal muscle stretching exercises.

Further Reading

Brukner P, Khan K (2006). *Clinical Sports Medicine* (3rd edn). Sydney: McGraw-Hill.

England and Wales Cricket Board (ECB) (2011). *ECB Fast Bowling Directives*. Available at: http://www.ecb.co.uk/ecb/publications/ecb-fast-bowling-directives,100,BP.html (accessed 6 June 2011).

Case 33

A 28-year-old female runner presented to the sport and exercise medicine clinic with left anterior knee pain. She had started regular running 6 weeks previously as she was preparing for the London Marathon that was taking place in 4 months. At presentation, she was running three times a week, up to 5 km at a time. Prior to this she had not engaged in regular physical activity. The onset of the knee pain was insidious but had become gradually worse over the preceding 4 weeks. The pain was notably worsened on running and she had noted stiffness after driving. She had not suffered any injury to the left knee.

On examination, she was noted to over-pronate at the subtalar joint of the left foot. She had weak hip abductors and reduced flexibility of her hip flexors which was more pronounced on the left side. She had little quadriceps muscle bulk. The inferior patellar facets were tender to palpation. The patellar tendon was non-tender. Joint range of motion was normal and pain free. Examination of the knee ligaments and menisci was normal. Hip joint examination was normal.

Questions

1. What are the main differential diagnoses of anterior knee pain associated with physical activity?
2. What is the diagnosis in this case?
3. What is the underlying pathophysiology of this condition?
4. What factors may contribute to development of this condition?
5. How would you manage this condition?

Answers

1. What are the main differential diagnoses of anterior knee pain associated with physical activity?

Anterior knee pain is a common complaint amongst inactive and physically active subjects. The common causes of anterior knee pain in the physically active are:

◆ patello-femoral pain syndrome (PFPS)

◆ patellar tendinopathy

◆ fat pad impingement

◆ quadriceps tendinopathy

◆ Osgood–Schlatter disease and osteochondritis dissecans (young patients)

◆ referred pain from the hip joint (especially slipped capital femoral epiphysis in younger subjects).

2. What is the diagnosis in this case?

The likely diagnosis in this case is PFPS. This is a term used to describe all peripatellar and retropatellar pain in the absence of other pathology. Clinical examination should be sufficient to exclude other potential causes of anterior knee pain and further investigations are not necessary.

3. What is the underlying pathophysiology of this condition?

The exact cause and origin of PFPS is currently unknown. It is thought that multiple structures in and around the knee joint can contribute to the pain. When the knee is at full extension the patellar is lateral to the trochlea of the femur. During knee flexion, the patella moves medially to lie in the intercondylar notch of the femur. This brings it into contact with a larger surface area, offsetting the increased load within the patello-femoral joint (PFJ). Dysfunctional movement of the patella during flexion will result in alterations in intra-articular pressure. This may cause pain when combined with increased loading on the PFJ, for example when running or climbing stairs.

4. What factors may contribute to development of this condition?

Any factor that increases PFJ load can contribute to the development of PFPS; there are intrinsic and extrinsic factors. Extrinsic factors include increases in training frequency, poor shock-absorbent footwear, and running on hard surfaces. Intrinsic factors relate to suboptimal patellar movement which include the following:

◆ Patellar position

◆ Decreased gluteus medius strength and endurance

◆ Weak hip flexors

- Inadequate muscle flexibility in the hip flexors, hamstrings, and soleus/gastrocnemius complex
- Increased subtalar pronation
- Tight lateral structures of the knee
- Delayed onset of vastus medialis obliterans (VMO) muscle contraction compared with the vastus lateralis muscle
- Increased knee valgus.

5. How would you manage this condition?

PFPS is best treated with an individually tailored programme addressing intrinsic and extrinsic factors. Pain can be treated with ice, simple analgesics, and taping of the patella. Extrinsic factors should be addressed and patients advised to have relative rest from aggravating activities and to engage in non-exacerbating exercise such as swimming. Any training errors should be corrected and patients educated regarding footwear and running surfaces. Strength and stretching programmes should be developed, guided by the intrinsic factors identified. In strengthening programmes, particular attention should be paid to VMO muscle, hip abductors, and hip external rotator muscles. Hip flexors, hamstrings, and soleus/gastrocnemius complex muscle flexibility should be improved. Orthotics may be used in patients who over-pronate. The patient should be advised that it may take up to 12 weeks before they see the benefits of the exercise programme.

Further reading

Crossley K, Cook J, Cowan S, McConnell J (2006). Anterior knee pain. In: Brukner P, Khan K (eds). *Clinical Sports Medicine* (3rd edn). Sydney: McGraw-Hill; pp. 506–37.

Fagan V, Delahunt E (2008). Patellofemoral pain syndrome: a review on the associated neuromuscular deficits and current treatment options. *Br J Sports Med*; **42**: 789–95.

Case 34

A 72-year-old man had been under the care of the rheumatology department for 3 years with a polyarthritis involving his hands, knees, and ankles. The hands had been especially uncomfortable across the wrists and MCPs. The blood tests had been normal apart from an elevated CRP of 25–30 mg/L. A diagnosis of RA had been made, although the RF and ACPA tests were negative, X-rays did not demonstrate erosions, and there was no family history of RA or autoimmunity.

The past medical history included chronic bronchitis, probably smoking-related, although he had stopped smoking 18 years previously. Medications included simvastatin for elevated cholesterol and low-dose aspirin. His RA was treated with sulfasalazine 2 g daily for 2.5 years.

At his routine follow-up appointment he was noted to have a red left eye. He also described pain on the pinnae of both ears such that he had difficulty sleeping on his side. Examination revealed that the pinnae were swollen, red, and tender. The ear lobes were normal. An ophthalmology assessment confirmed scleritis in the left eye. The rest of the ocular examination was normal. At this point, the ESR was 55 mm/h and the CRP was 48 mg/L.

The diagnosis was revised, the sulfasalazine was discontinued, and he was commenced on 40 mg of prednisolone, to which there was a prompt positive response in all the clinical and laboratory parameters.

Questions

1. What is the diagnosis and why?
2. What is the pathophysiology of this condition?
3. What clinical features might occur in patients with this diagnosis?
4. What is the treatment?
5. What is the prognosis?

Answers

1. What is the diagnosis and why?

The diagnosis is chronic relapsing polychondritis (RP). This is a rare chronic disorder of cartilage characterized by recurrent episodes of inflammation involving cartilaginous structures, predominantly those of the ears, nose, and laryngotracheobronchial tree. Other affected structures include the eyes, cardiovascular system, peripheral joints, skin, middle and inner ear, and CNS. RP may occur at any age, however, the disease usually has an onset during the fifth decade of life. There is no gender difference, but it is probably more common in Caucasians (few data exist).

2. What is the pathophysiology of this condition?

The aetiology is unknown. Evidence for an autoimmune pathogenesis includes the presence of infiltrating T cells, antigen–antibody complexes in affected cartilage, cellular and humoral responses against collagen type II and other collagen antigens, and the observation that immunosuppressive regimens usually suppress the disease. The level of antibodies to type II collagen present during the acute episodes correlates with the severity of the episode. Treatment with prednisolone is associated with a decrease in antibody titre. An autoimmune aetiology is further supported by the high prevalence of other autoimmune disorders found in these patients: 25–35% of patients have a concurrent autoimmune disease, and the associations include thyroid disease, vasculitis, RA, SLE, Sjögren's syndrome, and IBD. Familial clustering has not been observed. Susceptibility for developing RP is increased slightly by the HLA-DR4 haplotype.

Several reports have linked relapsing RP with malignancy. It is thought to be paraneoplastic in these cases, most often haematological, but solid tumours have been described.

3. What clinical features might occur in patients with this diagnosis?

As in this case, the non-specific and episodic nature of RP may result in delay in diagnosis. General signs and symptoms of constitutional upset with fever and weight loss are common. Diagnostic criteria for RP were first proposed by McAdam and colleagues and have been modified several times.

The criteria are as follows (three of the six clinical features are necessary for diagnosis):

◆ bilateral auricular chondritis
◆ non-erosive seronegative inflammatory polyarthritis
◆ nasal chondritis
◆ ocular inflammation
◆ respiratory tract chondritis
◆ audiovestibular damage.

Auricular chondritis occurs in 85–95% and maybe unilateral or bilateral, sparing the lobules.

◆ The ear cartilage softens and collapses forwards. The external auditory canal can collapse after one or more episodes.

◆ Nodularity of the auricle may develop.

◆ Calcification occurs in 40% of patients.

The arthritis is non-erosive and seronegative, and is a polyarthritis in 52–85% of patients. The acute onset of an inflamed joint may mimic a crystal arthropathy.

Nasal chondritis occurs in 48–72% of patients and the classical saddle-nose deformity may develop in long-standing disease.

Ocular sequelae occur in 50–65% and are related to the episodic inflammation of the uveal tract, conjunctivae, sclerae, and/or corneas.

◆ The most common conditions are episcleritis (39%) and scleritis (14%).

◆ Eyelid oedema, iritis, and retinopathy are found in 9% of patients, and 5% have ocular muscle paresis or optic neuritis.

◆ Ulcerative keratis is found in 4% of patients and has been associated with perforation and endophthalmitis.

Respiratory tract involvement affects 40–56% of patients. Tenderness to palpation may occur over the anterior trachea or thyroid cartilage. Chondritis weakens the tracheal cartilage rings, resulting in wheezing, dyspnoea, cough, and hoarseness. The upper airways can become stenosed and replaced by collapsible fibrotic tissue. Airways superior to the thoracic inlet collapse upon inspiration, and airways below the thoracic inlet collapse upon expiration, therefore both inspiratory stridor and expiratory wheezing may be noted. Inflammation and swelling of the glottis, larynx, and subglottic tissues may require tracheostomy. Acute inflammation of the distal airways can lead to obstruction and recurrent pneumonia.

Audiovestibular derangements occur in 46–50% of patients. Sudden loss of hearing is usually permanent, but tinnitus, nausea, vomiting, and vertigo may subside. In some patients, hearing loss is attributed to vasculitic damage to cranial nerve VIII.

Other systems that may be involved include the following:

◆ Cardiovascular
  • Affects 24% of patients.
  • Aortic and mitral valve regurgitation, aortic aneurysm, aortitis, aortic thrombosis, pericarditis, first- to third-degree heart block, and myocardial infarction due to ostial stenosis of a coronary artery or arteries have been reported.

◆ Skin
  • Skin lesions are found in 17–39% of patients.
  • Specific lesions are limited to erythema and oedema overlying the inflamed cartilaginous structures.
  • Other non-specific skin lesions have been reported including Sweet's syndrome, aphthous ulcers, urticarial vasculitis, and panniculitis.

- MAGIC syndrome—mouth and genital ulcers with inflamed cartilage. This is characterized by an overlap of RP with BD.
- Central nervous system
  - CNS manifestations are rare and related to a small- and/or medium-vessel vasculitis.
- Renal
  - 22% of patients have evidence of glomerulonephritis based on renal biopsy or the presence of microhaematuria and proteinuria.
  - Patients with renal damage are older and more likely to have extra-renal vasculitis and arthritis.
  - The biopsy findings include segmental necrotizing glomerulonephritis with or without crescents, interstitial lymphocytic infiltrates, interstitial fibrosis, active tubulitis, and glomerulosclerosis.

4. What is the treatment?

No controlled trials of therapy for RP have been published. The aim of treatment is to relieve symptoms and preserve the integrity of cartilaginous structures.

Steroids are the mainstay of treatment. Prednisolone (20–60 mg/day) is administered in the acute phase and is tapered for maintenance. Severe flares may require 80–100 mg/day. Most patients require a low daily dose of steroid for maintenance. However, intermittent administration of high doses only during flares of the condition can be successful.

Other medications reported to control symptoms and delay progression of the disease include dapsone (25–200 mg/day), azathioprine, methotrexate, cyclophosphamide, and ciclosporin. Leflunomide has also been used with some success. There are case reports describing successful treatment with the TNF-α inhibitors infliximab, etanercept, and adalimumab. Anakinra, an interleukin 1 receptor antagonist, and rituximab have also shown benefit. NSAIDs are not effective.

Medical care must include assessment for and treatment of other autoimmune disorders.

As RP is a complex multisystem condition it requires a team approach to management including dermatologists, ophthalmologists, cardiologists, neurologists, and plastic surgeons. Surgical care may include tracheostomy, permanent tracheostomy placement, tracheal stent placement, aortic aneurysm repair, cardiac valve replacement, and saddle-nose deformity repair.

5. What is the prognosis?

A survival rate of 94% at 8 years has been reported, but this may be shorter if there is associated systemic vasculitis.

The most frequent causes of death are infection secondary to corticosteroid treatment or respiratory compromise (10–50% of deaths result from airway complications), systemic vasculitis, and malignancy unrelated to RP.

Although the life expectancy in all patients with RP is decreased compared with age- and sex-matched healthy individuals, patients with renal involvement have a significantly lower age-adjusted life expectancy.

Complications of RP such as saddle nose, systemic vasculitis, laryngotracheo-bronchial stricture, arthritis, and anaemia in patients younger than 51 years portend a poorer prognosis than in age-matched patients with RP without complications. Among patients older than 50 years, only anaemia is associated with a poorer prognosis. Renal involvement is a poor prognostic factor at all ages.

Further reading

Letko E, Zafirakis P, Baltatzis S, Voudouri A, Livir-Rallatos C, Foster CS (2002). Relapsing polychondritis: a clinical review. *Semin Arthritis Rheum*; **31**: 384–95.

McAdam LP, O'Hanlan MA, Bluestone R, Pearson CM (1976). Relapsing polychondritis: prospective study of 23 patients and a review of the literature. *Medicine (Baltimore)*; **55**: 193–215.

Priori R, Conti F, Pittoni V, Valesini G (1997). Relapsing polychondritis: a syndrome rather than a distinct clinical entity? *Clin Exp Rheumatol*; **15**: 334–5.

Trentham DE, Le CH (1998). Relapsing polychondritis. *Ann Intern Med*; **129**: 114–22.

Case 35

A 29-year-old man was referred to the rheumatology outpatient department with a 2-month history of cramps and muscular aching in his arms and thighs. He was normally healthy, apart from hay fever in the summer. He worked as a forklift-truck driver in a warehouse. He had no significant family history, apart from non-insulin-dependent diabetes in his father, and his only travel in the preceding 5 years had been to Europe. He exercised regularly and had run a marathon 3 months previously. Following the marathon, he recalled having an upper respiratory infection and cough which had settled completely with a 7-day course of amoxicillin. On direct questioning, he denied rash or Raynaud's phenomenon.

Clinical examination revealed slight tenderness of the arms and thighs. The tissue felt taut, tethered, and oedematous. His face, neck, and torso were normal. Nailfolds were normal. Respiratory examination, muscle power, and neurological examination were normal.

Investigations showed the following:

- Hb 14.6 g/L; WBC 5.8 × 10^9/L; eosinophil count 1.2 × 10^9/L; platelets 335 × 10^9/L
- ESR 45 mm/h; CRP 16.3 mg/L
- Biochemistry normal
- CPK 321 IU/mL
- Thyroid function normal.

Questions

1. Give a differential diagnosis for this man's symptoms.
2. What radiological investigations may be helpful?
3. What single test would be required to secure the diagnosis?
4. What treatment modalities may be useful?
5. What is the prognosis?

Answers

1. Give a differential diagnosis for this man's symptoms

Potential causes of skin tethering in this case include:

◆ scleroderma

◆ overlap connective tissue disease with features of scleroderma

◆ scleredema

◆ eosinophilic fasciitis (EF)

◆ eosinophilia–myalgia syndrome.

The absence of Raynaud's phenomenon is an important negative finding and would be against the diagnosis of scleroderma or a connective tissue disease. Furthermore, the normal nailfolds and a normal facial appearance without any skin tightening are against a diagnosis of scleroderma. An autoantibody profile may be helpful in diagnosing an autoimmune disease, but if it were negative, it would not exclude the diagnosis.

Occasionally there can be muscle pains and a brawny oedema of the soft tissues in the early stages of dermatomyositis. The normal muscle power and muscle enzymes would be against this diagnosis in this case. Viral or autoimmune polymyositis (see Case 29) may also present with muscle pains. The raised CRP suggests tissue injury, and therefore other mechanical or non-specific causes of aching such as fibromyalgia (see Case 27) are unlikely.

Scleredema is characterized by a woody non-pitting induration of the skin with mild erythema. Although regarded as a benign self-limiting skin disease, scleredema may be persistent and involve the viscera. A skin biopsy will demonstrate increased collagen in affected sites. Involvement of the skin over the joints may cause limited range of motion. Scleredema on the face can result in difficulty in opening the eyes and the mouth. Although rare, extensive truncal involvement may cause restrictive lung disease. Unlike scleroderma, the tongue may be involved in scleredema, resulting in dysarthria and difficulty with mastication and tongue protrusion. The absence of oesophageal involvement distinguishes scleredema from scleroderma. Cardiac involvement is rare in scleredema but may result in cardiomyopathy. Fifty per cent of scleredema cases occur in individuals younger than 20 years of age. Scleredema can be categorized into three clinical subgroups. Each has a different history, course, and prognosis.

◆ Group 1, scleredema adultorum, includes scleredema after acute respiratory infection. Patients have a history of a preceding febrile illness, particularly an upper respiratory tract streptococcal infection. The onset of the skin lesions is rapid, and the condition usually clears spontaneously in 6 months to 2 years. The duration is not affected by the use of antibiotics. The term scleredema adultorum is considered by some to be a misnomer because most paediatric patients fall into this group. The patient described in this case may fit this picture in view of his history of respiratory illness. However, he did not have the typical pattern of skin involvement: there was no torso involvement and the skin induration was more distal than proximal. A skin and fascial biopsy would be helpful.

♦ Group 2 includes scleredema patients whose disease occurs insidiously with no preceding illness. This group is associated with a monoclonal gammopathy and myeloma.

♦ Group 3, scleredema diabeticorum, is scleredema associated with diabetes mellitus and includes patients with pre-existing diabetes, which is typically adult in onset and insulin dependent. This disorder tends to occur more often in males, and this subgroup of patients typically experience a more protracted course that is refractory to therapy. As in group 2, the onset of skin lesions is insidious. The upper back typically demonstrates erythema and induration, and a pebbled appearance may develop.

EF is a rare localized fibrosing disorder of the fascia described by Shulman in 1974. The aetiology and pathophysiology are unclear. Current understanding of the disease relies on a few case series and multiple case reports. Fascial thickening in the setting of eosinophilia, elevated ESR, and hypergammaglobulinaemia are key elements of the syndrome (Fig. 35.1). Visceral involvement is generally absent. However, an association with several haematological diseases is recognized and it frequently carries a poor prognosis. A number of possible triggers have been reported. There is a preceding history of vigorous exercise or trauma in 30–50% of patients. Multiple drugs have also been implicated, including simvastatin, atorvastatin, and phenytoin. Several cases have been associated with positive *Borrelia* serology.

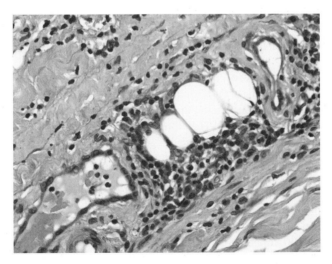

Fig. 35.1 (See also Plate 15) Fascial sclerosis with lymphocytic, plasma cell, and eosinophilic infiltration. (Reproduced from Servy A *et al.* (2010) *Patholog Res Int*; © 2011 Amandine Servy *et al.*)

Eosinophilia–myalgia syndrome and toxic oil syndrome are two disorders that share common clinical and histopathological features with EF, including peripheral eosinophilia. In contrast with EF, these two conditions present in epidemic form and appear to be almost universally toxin-associated, as in the case of the Spanish toxic oil syndrome in 1981.

2. What radiological investigations may be helpful?

MRI is the imaging modality of choice and shows characteristic findings of fascial thickening, abnormal signal intensity, and contrast enhancement. MRI may aid in diagnosis, locating a biopsy site, and monitoring the response to treatment. Although ultrasonography has not been used frequently or studied in EF, one case report has shown that it can aid early diagnosis.

3. What single test would be required to secure the diagnosis?

The diagnosis is that of eosinphilic fasciitis. The definitive diagnosis requires a full-thickness incisional skin biopsy. The specimen should include the skin, fat, fascia, and superficial muscle in continuity. Biopsy is especially important in an atypical presentation.

The hallmarks of EF are inflammation, oedema, thickening, and sclerosis of the fascia. In the acute phase, lymphocytes, plasma cells, histiocytes, and eosinophils infiltrate deep fascia and an adjacent subcutis layer. Distribution of the eosinophils in the fascia may be focal, and a close relationship appears to exist between blood and tissue eosinophilia. In the deeper portions of the panniculus, a similar infiltrate is found in the fibrous septa and at the periphery of the fat lobules. Deep in the fascia, the inflammatory infiltrate can extend into the epimysium, perimysium, and endomysium. In addition, vascular cuffing with lymphocytes and plasma cells is often seen.

As the disease progresses, the inflammatory changes are replaced by generalized sclerosis and thickening of the fascia and adjacent tissue layers. *In situ* hybridization with specific cDNA demonstrates that lesional fibroblasts produce excess collagen and display elevated TGF-β. Therefore the pathogenesis appears to involve the concomitant increase in the expression of genes for TGF-β and extracellular matrix proteins in fibroblasts in the affected tissues.

4. What treatment modalities may be useful?

When considering medical therapies for EF, especially second-line agents, it should be borne in mind that up to a third of cases may resolve spontaneously.

Systemic corticosteroids are the initial therapeutic agent of choice. Prednisolone is typically used in doses ranging from 20 to 100 mg/day. Response is considered satisfactory with reduction in oedema, improvement in skin thickening, resolution of carpal tunnel syndrome (which may also be a feature), and a gradual decrease in joint contracture. Eosinophilia and inflammatory markers frequently resolve promptly after initiation of steroid therapy.

Disease-modifying or steroid-sparing agents may be useful in persistent or steroid-resistant cases. Treatment numbers are small, and controlled trials are lacking. Case reports detail the use of multiple additional agents including antihistamines, cimetidine, hydroxychloroquine, azathioprine, ciclosporin, dapsone, tacrolimus, methotrexate, griseofulvin, ketotifen, and interferon-α, with varying rates of response. Recent data suggest that anti-TNF-α agents may also be beneficial.

Physical therapy should be initiated to improve joint mobility and to decrease contractures. Surgical release has been used in some cases to manage significant joint contractures.

5. What is the prognosis?

The loss of oedema is usually the first clinical sign of improvement and can occur within 4 weeks of commencing treatment. The skin becomes softer, but it can take 3–6 months before maximum reduction in induration and contractures is achieved. A degree of induration can remain even after many months of corticosteroid therapy. There is not a good correlation between clinical disease activity and laboratory findings. The eosinophilia and CRP usually return to reference ranges within 4–8 weeks, although the ESR and hypergammaglobulinaemia may remain abnormal for up to 12 weeks.

A recent retrospective review found that clinical factors associated with persistent fibrosis included the presence of morphea-like skin lesions, younger age at onset, truncal involvement, and presence of dermal fibrosclerosis on histopathological specimens. The development of aplastic anaemia is a rare and serious complication.

Further reading

Lakhanpal S, Ginsburg WW, Michet CJ, Doyle JA, Moore SB (1988). Eosinophilic fasciitis: clinical spectrum and therapeutic response in 52 cases. *Semin Arthritis Rheum*; **17**: 221–31.

Servy A, Clérici T, Malines C, Le Parc JM, Côté JF (2011). Eosinophilic fasciitis: a rare skin sclerosis. *Patholog Res Int*; 716935.

Case 36

A 71-year-old woman presented to the rheumatology clinic with a painful ulcer of the right lower leg. She reported worsening fatigue over the previous 6 months and had lost about half a stone in weight over this time. She was known to have RF-positive rheumatoid arthritis, diagnosed 40 years previously. Her disease had been difficult to control and she had undergone multiple joint replacements and spinal stabilization. She had had leg ulcers in the past but was concerned that this ulcer was not healing, was intensely painful, and often bled.

On examination, there was a large circumferential ulcer on the medial aspect of the right lower leg, extending upwards from the ankle (Fig. 36.1). The ulcer was oozing blood.

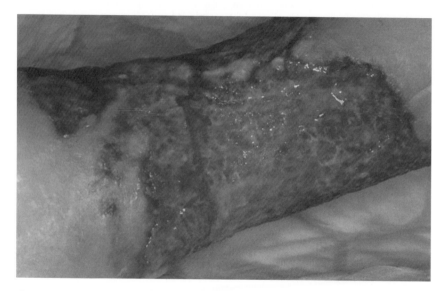

Fig. 36.1 (See also Plate 16) Circumferential leg ulcer.

Investigations showed the following:

- Hb 9.5 g/L; WCC 6.59 × 10⁹/L (neutrophils 4.81, lymphocytes 0.92); platelets 231 × 10⁹/L; MCV 83.8 fL
- Sodium 139 mmol/L; potassium 4.1 mmol/L
- Urea 9.3 mmol/L; creatinine 84 µmol/L
- CRP 54 g/L; ESR 46 mm/h.

Questions—Part 1

1. What are the possible causes of leg ulcers in patients with RA?
2. What is the approach to management of RA leg ulcers?

Answers

1. What are the possible causes of leg ulcers in patients with RA?

Patients with RA are predisposed to the development of chronic leg ulcers, the aetiology of which is commonly multifactorial. Venous insufficiency, vasculitis, and impaired arterial circulation are the most common precipitating factors. Pyoderma gangrenosum is a rarer cause; local malignant change and infection are reasons why there might be a delay in healing.

Systemic rheumatoid vasculitis often presents as a cutaneous vasculitis with enlarging leg ulcers. Vasculitic ulcers are characteristically deep and painful, and are typically found in the areas of the medial and lateral malleoli. They are caused by a necrotizing vasculitis of medium-sized arteries which is histologically similar to that seen in PAN.

Venous ulcers commonly occur on the medial side of the leg. They are often associated with varicose eczema and local oedema. The surrounding skin is thickened with hyperkeratosis and there may be progression to chronic lipodermatosclerosis. In contrast to vasculitic ulcers, venous ulcers are relatively painless unless infected. Venous ulceration is due to chronic venous insufficiency and is largely a downstream effect of venous hypertension. Risk factors include varicose veins, deep vein thrombosis, previous trauma or surgery, advanced age, and immobility. In addition, chronic glucocorticoid use in RA patients further promotes ulceration by increasing skin fragility.

Arterial ulcers are usually found on the feet, particularly at pressure points such as the heel and toes. The ulcers appear 'punched out' with a well-defined border, and are characteristically painful. The patient will usually have other features of arterial insufficiency including pale cool feet and leg pain on exertion or elevation. Arterial ulcers occur as a result of arterial insufficiency caused by atherosclerosis of the lower-limb arteries. Patients will have an impaired ankle–brachial pressure index (ABPI) on clinical assessment.

In pyoderma gangrenosum, lesions often progress quickly and may start at the site of a minor tissue injury, often first appearing as a small red papule or nodule. Breakdown of the skin then results in the formation of painful ulcers. Classically, they have a well-defined border and are violet or blue in colour. As the lesions enlarge, the edge may be undermined and the surrounding skin can become indurated. Several ulcers may occur at the same time.

In the case history described, the painful non-healing ulcer in a patient with long-standing seropositive RA raises the possibility of underlying rheumatoid vasculitis. The additional constitutional symptoms of fatigue and weight loss are typical. Rheumatoid vasculitis usually occurs in long-standing RA after the inflammatory arthritis has subsided and patients are left with widespread joint destruction. Patients are usually positive for rheumatoid factor and have rheumatoid nodules. The onset of vasculitis is usually associated with constitutional symptoms. However, symptoms such as fatigue, myalgia, and weight loss are non-specific and may be difficult to interpret in these debilitated patients.

2. What is the approach to management of RA leg ulcers?

If there is no clinical evidence for a systemic vasculitis, ulcers should be managed in the same way as for any other patient with a leg ulcer. This may include moist saline dressings to help debride layers of slough from granulation tissue. In patients with exudative ulcers, occlusive hydrocolloid dressings are helpful. If there is no arterial insufficiency, compression bandages or stockings can help alleviate swelling due to venous stasis. If an ulcer fails to respond to these conservative measures, underlying rheumatoid vasculitis should be considered. Since treatment involves aggressive immunosuppression, the diagnosis is best first confirmed by biopsy of the lesion.

Questions—Part 2

3. What different types of rheumatoid vasculitis occur?

4. What are the principles of treatment of rheumatoid vasculitis?

5. Discuss the role of cyclophosphamide therapy for rheumatoid vasculitis.

Answers

3. What different types of rheumatoid vasculitis occur?

Rheumatoid vasculitis affects a range of blood vessel types. These include medium-sized muscular arteries, arterioles, and venules. Like other forms of systemic vasculitis, there is destructive inflammation of the vessel wall, which leads to vessel occlusion, tissue ischaemia, and necrosis. Many of the serious clinical manifestations are caused by a medium-sized vasculitis. However, sequelae of small-vessel involvement (e.g. purpura and petechiae) also occur.

Rheumatoid vasculitis can affect several organs, with skin, peripheral nerves, eyes, and heart most commonly involved. Deep cutaneous vasculitis is the most common and can also cause digital ischaemia and gangrene.

Peripheral nerve involvement is the result of a vasculitic neuropathy characterized by inflammation of the vasa nervorum which results in infarction of peripheral nerve fibres. Depending on the distribution of the inflammatory process, both mononeuritis multiplex and distal sensory or sensorimotor neuropathy can occur. Vasculitic neuropathy is typically rapid in onset and usually manifests as anaesthesia. If treated promptly, most patients have a gradual, although partial, return of nerve function.

Ocular manifestations of rheumatoid vasculitis include scleritis and peripheral ulcerative keratitis (PUK). While anterior scleritis is readily diagnosed on clinical examination, posterior scleritis is more subtle, and the symptoms of visual blurring and ocular tenderness are important clues. Both forms of scleritis are intensely painful. PUK is characterized by the development of ulceration near the corneo-scleral junction. Patients with PUK may develop the 'corneal melt' syndrome, caused by corneal keratolysis and subsequent perforation of the globe. This is a devastating complication as patients often abruptly lose vision in the affected eye.

Pericarditis is usually the earliest presentation of the cardiac manifestations of rheumatoid vasculitis. Arrhythmias can also occur, although it is often difficult to attribute these directly to vasculitis as patients often have other relevant comorbidities. Acute coronary syndromes resulting directly from coronary arteritis are unusual.

4. What are the principles of treatment of rheumatoid vasculitis?

Treatment should be guided by the type and severity of the organ damage.

Systemic rheumatoid vasculitis requires aggressive immunosuppressive therapy, and therefore it is important to consider comorbidity. Treatment regimens usually start with a combination of high-dose glucocorticoids and cyclophosphamide, and parallel those used in primary systemic vasculitis. Glucocorticoids are accepted as playing an important role in achieving early disease remission, despite a lack of robust trial data. Pulsed methylprednisolone is used initially and patients can be switched to oral prednisolone after a few days. Maintenance therapy includes azathioprine and/or methotrexate.

Treatment is guided by monitoring clinical response as well as inflammatory markers (CRP, ESR) and markers of organ function (e.g. urea, creatinine). Treatment is continued until disease remission is achieved.

5. Discuss the role of cyclophosphamide therapy for rheumatoid vasculitis

Cyclophosphamide is an established treatment of primary systemic vasculitides such as WG (see Case 23). Although no controlled trials have directly assessed the role of cyclophosphamide in the treatment of rheumatoid vasculitis, it is accepted as a first-line treatment. Of note, a small case series of rheumatoid vasculitis patients reported disease remission in all patients following daily oral cyclophosphamide therapy.

If cyclophosphamide cannot be used, azathioprine is an appropriate alternative with corticosteroids. Methotrexate has also been used, although there is limited evidence for its efficacy in rheumatoid vasculitis. The role of TNF inhibitors in rheumatoid vasculitis is not established. Case reports suggest positive outcomes, although it should be noted that randomized trials have shown no evidence for TNF inhibitors in WG or GCA.

Further reading

Heurkens AH, Westedt ML, Breedveld FC (1991). Prednisolone plus azathioprine treatment in patients with rheumatoid arthritis complicated by vasculitis. *Arch Intern Med*; **151**: 2249–54.

Oien RF, Hakansson A, Hansen BU (2001). Leg ulcers in patients with rheumatoid arthritis—a prospective study of aetiology, wound healing and pain reduction after pinch grafting. *Rheumatology*; **40**: 816–20.

Case 37

A 55-year-old woman with a history of seropositive erosive RA for 7 years attended the 'flare' clinic with a 1-day history of an acutely swollen, red, and painful right wrist, associated with increased fatigue and fever. She had been on weekly etanercept 50 mg for the previous year. In clinic 2 weeks previously, her joints were not inflamed and the DAS28 was 3.0.

Her medical history included a recent diagnosis of hypertension, for which bendroflumethiazide had been prescribed.

In clinic her temperature was 37.5°C. Examination of the right wrist revealed a hot tender swollen erythematous joint. Movement of the joint was restricted due to pain.

Investigations showed the following:

- Hb 11.5 g/dL; MCV 84 fL; WCC 11.1 × 10^9/L; neutrophils 9.0 × 10^9/L; platelets 320×10^9/L
- Sodium 135 mmol/L; potassium 3.0 mmol/L
- Urea 11 mmol/L; creatinine 120 μmol/L
- LFTs normal
- CRP 54 mg/L.

Three millilitres of turbid synovial fluid was aspirated from the joint and sent to the laboratory for analysis. The initial microscopy showed the following:

- WCC 60 000 μL; 80% polymorphonuclear leucocytes
- No organisms seen
- No crystals seen.

Questions

1. What is the differential diagnosis, based on history and examination?
2. Apart from joint aspiration, what other investigations might be useful?
3. What is the most common causative agent responsible for this patient's diagnosis?
4. How would you manage this patient?
5. What are the management strategies for patients who are on biological therapy?

Answers

1. What is the differential diagnosis, based on history and examination?

Septic arthritis

This is essential to consider in any patient presenting with an acute monoarthritis, but especially in patients with inflammatory joint disease on immunosuppressant treatment. The acuteness of the presentation with associated fever should suggest this as the most likely diagnosis.

A normal joint has several defence mechanisms which protect it from infection. Synovial fluid itself has bactericidal activity, and normal synovial cells have phagocytic activity. The inflammatory process that occurs in RA decreases these protective factors. Furthermore, already damaged synovium of patients with RA exhibits neovascularization and increased adhesion factors, which both increase susceptibility to bacteraemia.

Patients with RA may have a blunted response to infection—for example, no fever and a more insidious onset. Also, they can commonly present with a polyarticular distribution which can easily be mistaken for a flare. Such patients would be gravely ill.

RA flare

The acuteness and monoarticular presentation, in the context of a recent recording of relatively quiescent disease, make this less likely.

Crystal arthropathy

Gout or pseudo-gout may be considered, given the history of the thiazide diuretic and the mild degree of renal impairment. Her gender and the absence of a previous history of crystal arthropathy make it a less likely diagnosis than septic arthritis. However, polarized light microscopy on joint fluid analysis should be requested even in cases of suspected septic joints.

Other causes

Other less likely causes of an acute monoarthrosis to consider include trauma and a reactive arthritis.

2. Apart from joint aspiration, what other investigations might be useful?

Microbiology

Blood cultures are positive in ~50–70% of patients with septic arthritis. Consider addition of synovial fluid AFB testing and mycobacterium culture in any patient with a chronically infected joint and with immunosuppressant risk factors, such as anti-TNF therapy and HIV.

Plain X-ray of wrist

Plain X-rays are not useful in diagnosis of septic arthritis, but can be of benefit in recording baseline findings especially in a patient with RA. They also may show chondrocalcinosis or any evidence of trauma.

Early plain radiograph findings of septic joints may demonstrate soft tissue swelling and widened joint space due to a joint effusion. Progression of sepsis usually leads to articular cartilage destruction, seen initially as the loss of visualization of the white cortical line of the joint surface, followed by poorly defined marginal erosions and joint-space narrowing. In more chronic cases superimposed osteomyelitis, seen as a periosteal reaction, and bone destruction may develop.

Other imaging

Ultrasound scanning is of limited value as a diagnostic tool in patients with suspected septic joints. However, it is a sensitive tool for detecting joint effusions and thereby facilitating guided-needle aspiration for synovial fluid. This is useful in smaller joints where direct aspiration may be difficult.

MRI is a sensitive tool which is increasingly used in the evaluation and management of septic joints. The presence of a joint effusion, synovial enhancement, and perisynovial soft tissue oedema is closely correlated with diagnosis of a septic joint. These findings are usually evident within 24 hours of onset of infection. Bone marrow signal changes can indicate associated osteomyelitis, the presence of which may guide surgical intervention as well as duration of antibiotic therapy.

Other investigations

A serum urate level is usually of little value in a patient with acute gout.

3. What is the most common causative agent responsible for this patient's diagnosis?

Staphyloccocus aureus, streptococci, and *Neisseria gonorrhoea* are bacteria with a high affinity for synovium because of their specific adherence factors and toxin-related mechanisms. Organisms most commonly invade the joint via haematogenous spread, as well as via direct inoculation and contiguous spread from periarticular infected tissue.

Staphylococcus aureus accounts for more than 80% of cases of septic arthritis in patients with RA. It also causes the vast majority of cases of bacterial arthritis in non-RA adults and children above the age of 2 years. *S.aureus* has a variety of tissue adhesion receptors, termed microbial surface components recognizing adhesive matrix molecules (MSCRAMM). These mediate adherence to extracellular joint components, for example fibronectin, elastin, and hyaluronic acid. Invasion of the joint by *S.aureus* is followed by release of chondrocyte proteases by the organism. This, combined with the cytokine synthesis from the host's polymorphonuclear leucocytes, results in rapid cartilage degradation. Irreversible subchondral bone loss can occur within days.

S.aureus is also the most common organism implicated in prosthetic joint infections. MSCRAMMS are implicated in the adherence of the bacteria to implanted medical devices such as prosthetic joints.

Prosthetic joint infections are associated with a high morbidity. The pathogenesis of prosthesis infections is related to the development of biofilms. Biofilm formation is particularly associated with *S.aureus*, coagulase-negative staphylococci, and *Pseudomonas aeruginosa*. Having adhered to the surface of the prosthesis, the bacteria cluster together. Because of a lack of metabolic substances and an accumulation of waste products, the organisms enter a slow-growing state. This results in significant resistance to growth-dependent antimicrobial agents. Furthermore, the synthesis of a polymeric matrix of saccharides, or glycocalyx, protects the bacteria from the host's defences and antimicrobial therapy. This explains the indolent nature of prosthetic infections and the difficulties in eradicating the infection.

Prosthetic joint infections can be classified according to the route of infection and according to onset of symptoms after infection. Routes of infection include perioperative direct contamination, haematogenous seeding from a distant focus of infection, and contiguous seeding from an adjacent focus of infection. Early prosthetic infections (i.e. within 3 months) are usually acquired during surgery and are associated with virulent organisms such as *S.aureus*. Delayed infections, occurring before 24 months, are also usually due to inoculation at the time of surgery but in association with less virulent organisms, such as coagulase-negative staphylococci. Late infection after 24 months is most frequently caused by haematogenous seeding.

The next most common organisms associated with septic arthritis are streptococci, particularly group A β-haemolytic streptococci and *Streptococcus pneumoniae*.

Septic arthritis caused by Gram-negative bacteria is more common in the very young, the elderly, the immunosuppressed, and intravenous drug abusers. Patients with HIV have a higher prevalence of joint infections than the normal population. Opportunistic organisms, such as mycobacteria and fungi, are more commonly implicated in this subset of patients.

Gonococcal arthritis needs to be in the differential diagnosis for younger sexually active individuals. The synovial fluid Gram stain and culture in gonococcal arthritis is less likely to be positive. *N.gonorrhoea* tends to cause less of a polymorphonuclear leucocyte response, thereby in part explaining the relatively smaller amount of joint destruction seen with this organism when compared with staphylococcal infection.

4. How would you manage this patient?

Management is multidisciplinary, including microbiology and orthopaedic advice.

Empirical antibiotic therapy should be commenced before the results of synovial fluid Gram stain or culture are available if there is a high index of suspicion of septic arthritis. Local policy and guidelines will influence choice of antibiotic.

The current BSR recommendations for empirical therapy are as follows.

◆ No risk factors for atypical organisms:
- intravenous flucloxacillin 2 g four times daily or intravenous clindamycin if penicillin allergic.

◆ High risk of Gram negative sepsis:
- second- or third-generation cephalosporin (i.e. cefuroxime or ceftriaxone).

◆ Suspected gonococcus:
- intravenous ceftriaxone.

The choice of antibiotic should be adjusted depending on synovial fluid culture and organism sensitivity. The microbiology team should be involved in decision-making.

Antibiotics are usually given intravenously for up to 2 weeks, and then orally for 4 weeks. However, this may vary depending on the response to therapy. Local hospital services may allow insertion of PICC lines and treatment on an outpatient basis via a home IV team or equivalent. The infected joint should ideally be drained to dryness, either via closed-needle approach or arthroscopically. The orthopaedic team should be involved early on, especially for hip or prosthetic joint sepsis.

There has been much debate in previous years about the benefits versus the risks of intra-articular steroid injections in patients with septic arthritis. Evidence from animal models suggests that the use of corticosteroids in addition to antibiotics could improve outcomes. One study in humans has also shown some benefit. A double-blind randomized placebo-controlled trial in 123 children compared intravenous dexamethasone and antibiotics with antibiotics alone. The addition of steroid reduced the duration and extent of joint damage.

The theory behind steroid use is based on the fact that bacterial antigens promote cytokine proliferation and activate chondrocyte proteases. Despite antibiotic treatment, inflammation may persist and intra-articular corticosteroid may limit this inflammatory damage. However, there is concern that steroid, especially early on, may mask the signs of infection and delay diagnosis.

5. What are the management strategies for patients who are on biological therapy?

Biological therapy should be stopped when there is infection. Unfortunately, there is currently little guidance and evidence on when biological therapy should be restarted after such an event.

BSR guidelines on anti-TNF prescribing state that joint sepsis within the previous 12 months is a contraindication to commencing biological therapy. This may be indefinite for an infected prosthetic joint, especially if the prosthesis is to be left *in situ*. This is based on clinical opinion, rather than strong trial evidence.

Data from the UK National Biologics register suggest that patients on anti-TNF are twice as likely to develop septic arthritis as those on DMARDS alone. The risk of septic arthritis is greatest in the first year of therapy, peaking at around 10 months.

Staphylococci are the most common organisms; *Listeria* and *Salmonella* were reported in the group treated with anti-TNF agents. Native and prosthetic joints were equally at risk in biologically treated patients.

In clinical practice the risks of anti-TNF therapy may need to be balanced with treating uncontrolled RA. In challenging situations the decision regarding restarting biological therapy earlier should involve discussing risks and benefits with the patient, as well as seeking opinion from microbiology and other experts.

Further reading

Coakley G, Mathews C, Field M, *et al.* (2006). BSR & BHPR, BOA, RCGP and BSAC guidelines for management of the hot swollen joint in adults. *Rheumatology*; **45**: 1039–41.

Galloway JB (2010). *Risk of Septic Arthritis in Patients with Rheumatoid Arthritis Treated with Anti-TNF therapy: Results from the BSR Biologics Register.* Available online at: https://www. rheumatology.org.uk/includes/documents/cm_docs/2010/o/op49_hall08a_thu_1400_ galloway.pdf.

Goldberg D (1998). Septic arthritis. *Lancet*; **351**: 197–202.

Lane S, Merry P (1999). Intra-articular corticosteroids in septic arthritis: beneficial or barmy? *Ann Rheum Dis*; **58**: 142–7.

Ledingham J, Deighton C (2005). Update on the British Society for Rheumatology guidelines for prescribing TNF blockers in adults with rheumatoid arthritis. *Rheumatology*; **45**: 157–63.

Odio CM, Ramirez T, Arias G, *et al.* (2003). Double blind, randomized, placebo controlled study of dexamethasone therapy for haematogenous septic arthritis in children. *Pediatr Infect Dis J*; **22**: 883–8.

Sakiniene E, Bremell T, Tarkowski A (1996). Addition of corticosteroids to antibiotic treatment ameliorates the course of experimental *Staphylococcus aureus* arthritis. *Arthritis Rheum*; **39**: 1596–1605.

Shirtliff ME, Mader JT (2002). Acute septic arthritis. *Clin Microbiol Rev*; **15**: 527–44.

Case 38

A 69-year-old woman with a 15-year history of seropositive rheumatoid arthritis (RA) presented with increasing neck pain and arm weakness. Over the preceding 9 months, she had experienced bilateral numbness and paraesthesia in her hands, suggestive of bilateral carpal tunnel syndrome. She denied lower-limb weakness or bowel or bladder disturbance. Her RA was treated with methotrexate and certolizumab, a pegylated anti-TNF-α monoclonal antibody. She had previously used many DMARDs, including hydroxychloroquine, sulfasalazine, gold, and ciclosporin, which had been ineffective in controlling her disease. In the past, she had undergone arthroplasty of her left shoulder, left knee, right hip, and bilateral forefoot.

Examination of her limbs revealed normal power and reflexes. Her plantar reflexes were not interpretable because of the previous forefoot surgery. Perineal sensation was intact.

The CT cervical spine and MRI spine of her neck are shown in Figs 38.1 and 38.2.

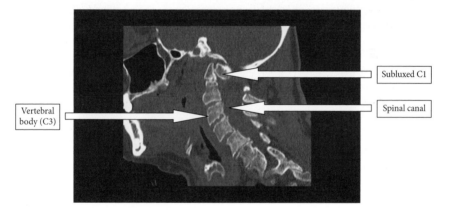

Vertebral body (C3)

Subluxed C1

Spinal canal

Fig. 38.1 CT scan of cervical spine.

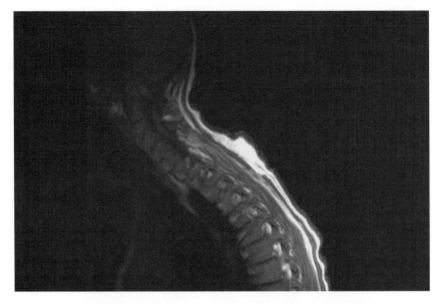

Fig. 38.2 MRI scan of neck.

Questions

1. Describe the radiographic findings. What abnormalities are indicated by the arrows?
2. What is the diagnosis?
3. What other spinal complications may occur in rheumatoid arthritis?
4. What conservative measures may be useful for rheumatoid neck disease?
5. What are the indications for neck surgery and what complications may occur?

Answers

1. Describe the radiographic findings. What abnormalities are indicated by the arrows?

Figure 38.1 demonstrates almost complete erosion of the odontoid peg with bony fragments behind the anterior arch of C1. There is severe posterolateral subluxation of C1 on C2 with no significant spinal canal narrowing. There is marked degenerative change at C4/5 and C6/7. The MRI confirms the odontoid peg erosion and subluxation at C0/1 and C1/2.

CT is the best modality to visualize bone and alignment abnormalities in the cervical spine as it can detect disc disease, fractures, tumours, infection, and stenosis.

MRI is used for evaluation of the spinal cord and neural components. It can detect subtle changes in bone, and is superior to CT in the evaluation of herniated discs, spinal stenosis, abscesses, osteomyelitis, tumours, or other masses near the spinal cord. MRI can demonstrate the presence of pannus (hyperplastic rheumatoid synovium) and its erosive effects on articular cartilage and local bone, as well as its resolution following immunosuppressant therapy. The relationship of the odontoid peg to the brainstem and oedematous changes in the cord can be evaluated. Further advantages of MRI are the absence of ionizing radiation and the infrequent need for intravenous contrast (gadolinium), the latter being much less allergenic than the iodinated contrast medium used in CT scanning.

The main indications for MRI imaging in rheumatoid cervical spine disease are:

- abnormal measurements of C1 to C2 on plain radiographs
- intractable suboccipital or cervical pain
- progressive or severe subluxation
- symptoms of cord compression
- vertebral artery compression.

2. What is the diagnosis?

The diagnosis is a cervical myelopathy secondary to erosion of the odontoid peg and transverse band of the cruciform ligament causing atlanto-axial instability and subluxation. In rheumatoid cervical spine disease, synovitis with pannus formation leads to erosion of ligaments, bones, and synovial joints (Fig. 38.3). Posterior movement of the odontoid peg may impinge on the upper cervical cord, particularly during neck flexion, with neurological sequelae. The rupture of the transverse ligament, and then the alar and apical ligaments, combined with erosion of the atlanto-axial (C1–2) joint leads to anterior atlanto-axial subluxation (AAS).

The usual symptoms of odontoid peg erosion are severe neck pain, pain or paraesthesia of the arms, limb weakness, sensory changes in the lower limbs, gait difficulties (spastic gait), and neck instability. In some patients, the first presentation is unexplained falls. The onset is often insidious and the symptoms are non-specific; therefore it is important to maintain a high index of suspicion for cervical spine involvement in rheumatoid patients.

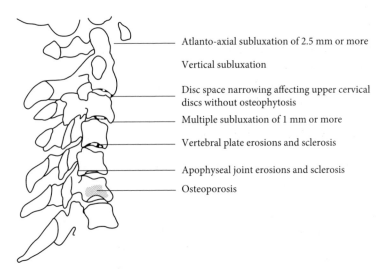

Atlanto-axial subluxation of 2.5 mm or more

Vertical subluxation

Disc space narrowing affecting upper cervical discs without osteophytosis

Multiple subluxation of 1 mm or more

Vertebral plate erosions and sclerosis

Apophyseal joint erosions and sclerosis

Osteoporosis

Fig. 38.3 Radiographic criteria for rheumatoid arthritis of the cervical spine. Reproduced from Winfield J, Cooke D, Brook A.S, Corbett M (1981). A prospective study of the radiological changes in the cervical spine in early rheumatoid disease. *Ann Rheum Dis*, **40**; 109–114 with permission from BMJ Publishing Group Ltd.

RA patients undergoing general anesthesia need careful pre-operative assessment and vigilant perioperative care to avoid cervical hyperextension and cervical cord injury during intubation.

Patients with damage at the occipito-cervical (O–C1) and C1–2 joints may present with high neck pain or occipital neuralgia, myelopathy, hydrocephalus, and rarely sudden death. The neurological sequelae can develop from a direct compressive effect on the spinal cord or from ischaemia. Compression of the spinal cord and eventually the brainstem can result from subluxation of the spine or from direct pressure by a synovial pannus.

3. What other spinal complications may occur in rheumatoid arthritis?

The spinal complications of RA can be subdivided as follows:

◆ cervical instability

◆ thoracolumbar vertebral abnormalities

◆ vertebral osteoporotic crush fracture.

Cervical instability

The most common patterns of cervical instability are:

◆ AAS—65% (Fig 38.4)

◆ ventral subluxation (VS)—20% (Fig. 38.5)

◆ subaxial subluxation—15–25%.

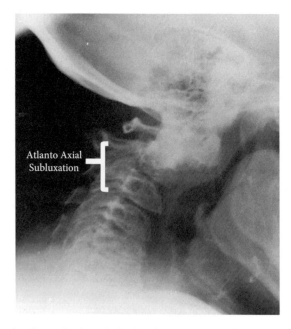

Fig. 38.4 Lateral radiograph of cervical spine demonstrating atlanto-axial subluxation.

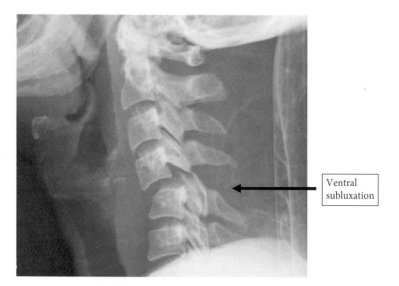

Fig. 38.5 Ventral subluxation.

The O–C1 and atlanto-axial C1–2 joints have a higher risk of subluxation than the lower cervical intervertebral joints as they are synovial joints. C1 anterior arch defects, dens erosions, or dens fractures sometimes cause posterior AAS. Although posterior or lateral AAS has a higher risk of cord compression, anterior AAS predominates. VS occurs secondary to cartilage and bone destruction at the O–C1 and C1–2 joints and is commonly preceded by AAS. This can present with a more severe neurological deficit and a poor prognosis.

Patients with RA and cervical disease should have plain radiographs of the cervical spine (in both flexion and extension) and a CT scan. MRI may also be useful to image the spinal cord.

Thoracolumbar vertebral abnormalities

Although the cervical spine is most commonly affected in RA, any synovial joint in the vertebral column can be affected. Involvement of the apophyseal joints and discovertebral junctions has been reported in the lumbar and thoracic spine. Intervertebral disc-space narrowing, irregularity of the subchondral margins of the vertebral bodies, erosion, and sclerosis can be seen on imaging.

Vertebral osteoporotic crush fracture

RA patients, particularly those with significant exposure to corticosteroids, are at risk of osteoporosis with subsequent wedge compression or fracture of the vertebral bodies. In addition, the resulting kyphosis which can be seen in these patients may lead to significant pain, deformity, and instability, and increase the technical difficulties of spinal surgery.

4. What conservative measures may be useful for rheumatoid neck disease?

The main aims in conservative treatment of rheumatoid neck disease are to relieve symptoms and prevent bone destruction.

- Patients require optimal DMARD therapy to control disease activity.
- Physiotherapy, in particular neck muscle strengthening exercises, and practical aids (e.g. a book rest when reading).
- A stiff neck collar can improve neck symptoms by restricting atlanto-axial movement, and is particularly useful for car journeys. Prolonged or continuous use of stiff neck collars can lead to weakness of neck muscles and is only recommended for patients with severe instability.
- Occipital nerve block may provide significant temporary relief for severe high cervical and occipital pain.

5. What are the indications for neck surgery and what complications may occur?

Whilst neurological examination can be difficult to interpret in patients with severe deforming RA of the feet, as in this patient, careful observation for evidence of neurological deterioration is important to detect early signs of myelopathy, as this may require urgent surgical intervention.

The main indications for cervical spinal surgery in RA are intractable pain, myelopathy, and AAS >8 mm.

Early prophylactic cervical spinal arthrodesis (fusion) with or without decompression can reduce the potential for paralysis. Surgical intervention in patients with significant cervical instability or subluxation without neurological deficit and minimal pain is controversial. Surgery in rheumatoid neck disease is complex and surgical site infection rates may be increased due to concomitant corticosteroid use, osteoporotic bone, and rheumatoid disease activity. Perioperative complications include vertebral artery injury, transient and persistent dysphagia or dyspnoea caused by pharyngeal obstruction, and neurological deterioration (e.g. paraparesis). Late postoperative complications include malunion and non-union.

Further reading

Calleja M (2009). *Rheumatoid Arthritis Spine Imaging.* http://emedicine.medscape.com/article/398955-overview.

Kauppi M (1996). Conservative treatment for rheumatoid cervical spine. *Lancet*; 347: 1695.

Moncur C, Williams HJ (1988). Cervical spine management in patients with rheumatoid arthritis. Review of the literature. *Phys Ther*; **68**; 509–15.

Neo M (2008). Treatment of upper cervical spine involvement in rheumatoid arthritis patients. *Mod Rheumatol*; **18**: 327–35.

Santavirta S, Kontinnen YT, Laasonen E, Honkanen V, Antti-Poika I, Kauppi M (1991). Ten year results of operations for rheumatoid cervical spine disorders. *J Bone Joint Surg Br*; **73**: 116–20.

Winfield J, Cooke D, Brook AS, Corbett M (1981). A prospective study of the radiological changes in the cervical spine in early rheumatoid disease. *Ann Rheum Dis*; **40**: 109–14.

Wollowick AL Casden AM, Kuflik PL, Neuwirth MJ (2007). Rheumatoid arthritis in the cervical spine: what you need to know. *Am J Orthop*; **36**: 400–6.

Zoma A, Sturrock RD, Fisher WD, Freman PA, Hamblen DL (1987). Surgical stabilisation of the rheumatoid cervical spine. A review of indications and results. *J Bone Joint Surg Br*; **69**: 8–12.

Case 39

A 35-year-old Caucasian male was referred to the rheumatology clinic with a 1-month history of knee and ankle pain, which had resolved by the time he was seen. He had previously been diagnosed with ulcerative colitis, requiring total colectomy in which a section of the small bowel, including the terminal ileum, had been resected to form an ileo-anal pouch anastomosis. He subsequently had recurrent episodes of pouchitis which were treated with steroids and antibiotics. Six years later he developed florid mouth ulceration.

The past medical history included a DVT at the age of 25, which had been treated with standard anticoagulation, and recurrent superficial thrombophlebitis. He had no history of genital ulcers. He had been treated for anterior uveitis with topical corticosteroids.

On examination, he had large mouth ulcers and tender erythematous lesions on the shins. He had a normal spine and neck examination.

Investigations showed the following:

- Hb 12.0 g/dL; MCV 85 fL; MCH 30 pg; WCC 6.2×10^9/L; platelets 214×10^9/L
- ESR 36 mm/h: CRP 50 mg/mL
- Normal renal and liver function tests
- Negative ANA, thrombophilia screen, and HLA B27.

Questions

1. What are the causes of severe oral ulceration?
2. Give the differential diagnoses. What is the most likely cause of his illness?
3. What are the clinical features of this condition?
4. What is the disease pathogenesis?
5. How should this condition be managed?

Answers

1. What are the causes of severe oral ulceration?

- Idiopathic recurrent oral stomatitis
- Nutritional (iron, vitamin B12, folate deficiencies)
- Infection (HIV, herpes simplex virus 1, CMV in immunocompromised patients)
- Drug reaction (nicorandil, bisphosphonates, NSAIDs)
- Gastrointestinal (ulcerative colitis, coeliac disease, Crohn's disease)
- Multisystem autoimmune disease (SLE, Reiter's disease, MAGIC)
- Dermatological (Sweet's syndrome, erythema multiforme, bullous skin disease)
- Haematological (cyclical neutropenia, lymphoma)
- Periodic fever syndromes: PFAPA (periodic fever, aphthous pharyngitis, and cervical adenopathy), familial Hibernian fever.

2. Give the differential diagnoses. What is the most likely cause of his illness?

- IBD-related spondyloarthropathy
- BD
- Reactive arthritis
- Sarcoidosis
- Connective tissue disease.

An IBD-related spondyloarthropathy may be considered in view of the development of joint pain in the lower limbs, inflammatory eye disease, and oral ulceration. However, it would not explain the history of thromboembolic disease, and is less likely given the negative HLA B27. A history of recent bowel or genitourinary infection may give rise to consideration of a reactive arthritis, but does not explain features such as florid mouth ulceration or DVT. Sarcoidosis may present with arthritis or arthralgia and erythema nodosum, and in rarer cases may involve the eye, but is unlikely to cause thromboembolism or inflammatory bowel lesions. A connective tissue disease may present with oral ulceration and arthralgia of the small joints, and be associated with thrombosis, but is unlikely in the presence of a negative ANA and thrombophilia screen. In view of the recurrent oral ulceration, arthralgia, erythema-nodosum-like lesions, inflammatory eye disease, and history of thrombosis, the most likely diagnosis is BD.

3. What are the clinical features of this condition?

Behçet's (pronounced Betjet's) disease (BD) is a multisystem chronic relapsing inflammatory disorder characterized by vasculitis of arteries and veins of all sizes in multiple organs. The International Study Group for Behçet's Disease diagnostic criteria published in 1990 include recurrent oral ulceration (three times in 1 year) and two of the following: recurrent genital ulcers, ocular inflammation, cutaneous lesions, and a positive pathergy test. There are no diagnostic laboratory tests but raised inflammatory markers may be present.

Oral ulceration is the most important diagnostic feature. Genital ulcers are the second most common manifestation and may be preceded by a papule or pustule and heal with scarring. Both oral and genital ulcers are painful.

Diagnostic cutaneous lesions are present in 80% of patients as papulopustular or acneiform lesions and erythema nodosum. Extragenital ulceration, superficial thrombophlebitis, and cutaneous vasculitis may also occur.

Pathergy, which is a cutaneous hypersensitivity to trauma, may be noted after venesection. It can be formally tested by the insertion of two large (20G) needles subcutaneously to 3 mm, a few centimetres apart, followed by examination by a physician after 48 hours. The test is positive if a papule or pustule develops at the site of insertion.

Gastrointestinal disease occurs in up to 30% of patients and can be difficult to differentiate from IBD. In this case, the original diagnosis of ulcerative colitis was probably incorrect and the patient was likely to have intestinal BD. This takes the form of mucosal ulceration and may be severe with large penetrating ulcers affecting any part of the gut, but most commonly located in the ileocaecal region.

Ocular inflammation is more frequent and severe in men, is bilateral in 85% cases, and may lead to blindness. It can take the form of anterior, posterior, or pan-uveitis, retinal vasculitis, optic neuritis, retinal vein occlusion, or the formation of a hypopyon. Posterior uveitis carries a particularly poor prognosis. This patient had a history of eye involvement and should be regularly screened by slit-lamp examination with aggressive management of eye disease.

Approximately 5% of patients with BD have neurological involvement. The CNS manifestations of BD may be parenchymal (80% of cases) or vascular. Cerebrovascular disorders include dural sinus thrombosis, arterial dissection, occlusions, and aneurysms. Peripheral neuropathy is uncommon.

Major vessel involvement may be due to inflammation or thrombosis and can involve both veins and arteries. Large vessel disease is predominantly venous, presenting as DVT or superficial thrombophlebitis. It may involve the superior and inferior vena cava. Budd–Chiari syndrome is caused by hepatic venous outflow obstruction within the liver or inferior vena cava and should be suspected in patients with BD who develop ascites and hepatosplenomegaly. Arterial or aortic rupture is the leading cause of sudden death in patients with BD. The presence of a pulmonary aneurysm in the setting of vasculitis is highly suggestive of BD. However, although major vessels may be involved, most manifestations are due to small-vessel disease.

Renal disease is most commonly caused by amyloidosis, but may also be caused by glomerulonephritis or tubulointerstitial nephritis.

Arthritis and arthralgia occur in 60% of patients as non-deforming oligoarticular disease affecting knees, ankles, and wrists. This is usually transient, lasting <2 months.

4. What is the disease pathogenesis?

BD prevalence and disease manifestations show regional and ethnic differences. BD is most common in Turkey, and its prevalence in the UK is much less at one in 100,000. It is a genetic disorder in which an environmental trigger, such as infection, is thought to stimulate autoinflammatory and autoimmune pathways, resulting in a systemic vasculitic and thrombotic disease. The presence of oral ulceration in 70% of patients with BD has led to the suggestion that oral microbial flora are implicated in the process.

BD is associated with the major histocompatibility complex (MHC) class I antigen HLA B5101 which is expressed in 60% of patients and increases the susceptibility to ocular disease. This contrasts with most classical autoimmune disorders which have an MHC class II association. Mutation of factor V Leiden is a common hereditary abnormality causing hypercoagulability and is associated with BD. Superficial thrombophlebitis is observed in combination with thrombosis in large veins, and clusters are observed with dural sinus thrombosis.

BD shares characteristics with the inherited autoinflammatory disorders (e.g. FMF). These involve the innate arm of the immune system in which recurrent inflammatory attacks occur with over-expression of proinflammatory cytokines. Symptoms include recurrent mucocutaneous lesions and non-deforming arthritis, but differ from BD by the presence of characteristic episodic fevers and serositis. Onset is usually in childhood.

BD also resembles an autoimmune disorder, since it involves increased T- and B-cell responses to heat-shock proteins, but it does not have the classical features of an autoimmune disease such as the presence of autoantibodies, a female preponderance, or association with other autoimmune diseases.

5. How should this condition be managed?

There have been no large randomized controlled trials of the management of BD. It is characterized by unpredictable exacerbations and remissions, but the exacerbations often become less severe and frequent with the passage of time. Therapy is guided by the clinical picture, and aggressive immunosuppression is given, where necessary, to limit organ damage.

Many patients can be managed symptomatically with mouthwashes and local steroids for oral ulceration and NSAIDs or colchicine for short episodes of arthritis. Corticosteroids, azathioprine, ciclosporin, interferon, and thalidomide can be used for more severe symptoms.

An aggressive approach is taken in treating inflammatory eye disease which may lead to blindness. Acute episodes are controlled with corticosteroids and cyclophosphamide or ciclosporin. Azathioprine has been shown to reduce or prevent recurrences of inflammatory eye disease and preserve visual acuity. Anti-TNF treatments, such as infliximab, have also been shown to be effective.

Thrombophlebitis is due to active inflammation of the endothelium with resultant thrombosis which does not embolize. Thus anticoagulation, which increases the risk of pulmonary haemorrhage in cases of pulmonary arteritis with aneurysm, is not necessary in such cases. However, anticoagulation will be required for cases of DVT or cerebral venous sinus thrombosis. Azathioprine is used to treat severe thrombophlebitis. Acute arteritis is treated with pulsed cyclophosphamide and steroids according to standard protocols for vasculitis.

Some patients go into complete remission, unlike in other autoimmune diseases. Patients with onset before 25 years of age have a poorer prognosis. Mortality and eye disease are increased among young males. This patient had intermittent courses of prednisolone and failed treatment with azathioprine and infliximab. He had a good response to ciclosporin 3 mg/kg/day but routine monitoring demonstrated a rise in creatinine from 50 to 70 μmol/L. Ciclosporin nephrotoxicity is an important cause of renal failure in patients with BD. Thalidomide 300mg daily was eventually successful in controlling his disease.

Further reading

Barnes CG (2006). Editorial. Treatment of Behçet's syndrome. *Rheumatology*; **45**: 245–7.

Direskeneli H (2006). Autoimmunity vs auto inflammation in Behçet's. Do we oversimplify a complex disorder? *Rheumatology*; **45**: 1461–5.

Keogan MT (2009). Clinical Immunology Review Series: an approach to the patient with recurrent orogenital ulceration, including Behçet's syndrome. *Clin Exp Immunol*; **156**: 1–11.

Sfikakis PP, Markomichelakis N, Alpsoy E, *et al.* (2007). Anti-TNF therapy in the management of Behçet's disease—review and basis for recommendations. *Rheumatology*; **46**: 736–41.

Yazici H, Fresko I, Yurdakul S (2007). Behçet's syndrome: disease manifestations, management, and advances in treatment. *Nat Clin Pract Rheumatol*; **3**: 148–55.

Case 40

A 21-year-old female Caucasian medical student presented to her GP with new-onset Raynaud's phenomenon affecting both hands. She described pain and colour changes in her left arm when she raised her arms above her head. During her medical student training she had discovered that the blood pressure was different when taken in each arm. Otherwise, she was systemically well. On examination, her blood pressure was 180/94 mmHg on the left and 110/60 mmHg on the right. There were no palpable pulses at her left wrist.

Investigations showed the following:

- Hb 10.2 g/L, MCV 82 fL, platelets 312 × 10⁹/L, WCC 6.3 × 10⁹/L
- ESR 18 mm/h, CRP <6 mg/L
- Negative ANA and thrombophilia screen
- MRA revealed occlusion of the left subclavian and proximal axillary arteries (Fig. 40.1)
- Urine analysis was normal.

A diagnosis of Takayasu's arteritis (TakA) was made and treatment was commenced.

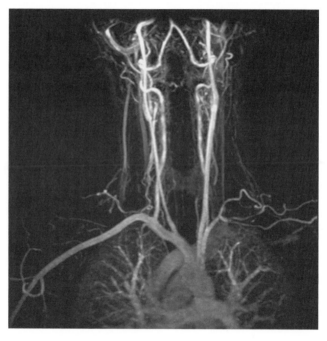

Fig. 40.1 Magnetic resonance arteriogram.

Questions

1. What are the similarities and differences between giant cell arteritis (GCA) and Takayasu's arteritis (TakA)?
2. Describe the course of TakA.
3. What are the treatment options for TakA?
4. Which imaging modalities may be useful in TakA?

Answers

1. What are the similarities and differences between giant cell arteritis (GCA) and Takayasu's arteritis (TakA)?

GCA and TakA are primary large-vessel vasculitides. Inflammation of the large arteries, such as the aorta and its major branches, occurs in a number of other disorders including Kawasaki disease, BD, rheumatoid arthritis, syphilis, and tuberculosis. GCA almost exclusively affects people over the age of 50 years and the incidence is highest in those who are aged 75–85 years. TakA classically affects young East Asian women, but occurs in both genders. The female-to-male ratio declines from East to West.

Both GCA and TakA present with signs of systemic inflammation: fever, malaise, myalgia, weight loss, and anaemia. GCA typically causes vasculitis of the extracranial branches of the aorta and spares intracranial vessels. Branches of the external and internal carotid arteries are particularly susceptible, leading to the classic manifestations of headache, scalp tenderness, and jaw claudication. TakA involves the large elastic arteries. Dilation, aneurysms, and thrombosis occur more frequently in TakA than GCA.

The histopathology of arterial lesions in both diseases may be indistinguishable, with a pan-arteritis and mononuclear infiltrates within all layers of the arterial wall. Typically activated T cells and macrophages are arranged in granulomata. The underlying aetiology is unknown for both diseases but evidence suggests T-cell-mediated autoimmunity. Circulating autoantibodies against aortic endothelial cells, which have been shown to induce aortic endothelial cell apoptosis, have been demonstrated. It is still unclear whether these antibodies are truly pathogenic and occur in a variety of other conditions where vascular inflammation is present.

2. Describe the course of TakA

TakA has an initial acute inflammatory phase and a chronic healed fibrotic phase with the development of vascular insufficiency. Clinical features are similarly divided into an early pre-pulseless systemic phase and a late occlusive phase characterized by diminished or absent pulses. In the early inflammatory phase, patients may show non-specific features of malaise, low-grade fever, night sweats, weight loss, arthralgia, fatigue, and rashes, including erythema nodosum. Investigations may show a normocytic anaemia and elevated inflammatory markers, but there are no specific disease markers. The presentation may overlap with those of infection or haematological malignancy, which should be excluded. However, clinical manifestations may be undetectable, as in this patient who presented with evidence of vessel damage and no history of inflammatory symptoms. Other conditions which may then be considered include coarctation of the aorta and Marfan's syndrome, ergotism, and neurofibromatosis, which have specific features enabling them to be differentiated from TakA.

The inflammatory phase may remit spontaneously, but usually progresses insidiously to the chronic phase. Vessel inflammation results in fibrosis, stenosis, and thrombus formation, and subsequent symptoms reflect end-organ ischaemia. Patients may notice easy fatiguability of the upper limbs, pain, and intermittent claudication. Many patients have diminished pulses or no pulses in the arm and blood pressure differences due to subclavian stenosis. Diminished pulses in the left upper limb are more frequent than on the right because of the vascular anatomy. There may be vascular bruits, particularly affecting the carotids and the subclavian and abdominal vessels. Patients with upper-limb vascular involvement may present as this woman did with Raynaud's phenomenon, ischaemic pain, and a difference in systolic blood pressure between arms. Patients with carotid artery involvement may present with neurological disease such as stroke, postural dizziness, seizures, and amaurosis. Aortic regurgitation results from dilatation of the ascending aorta. Hypertension most often reflects renal artery stenosis. Pulmonary vessel involvement may cause cough, dyspnoea, chest pain, and pulmonary hypertension.

3. What are the treatment options for TakA?

Initial treatment of TakA is induction of remission with corticosteroids followed by maintenance with a steroid-sparing agent to reduce arterial inflammation and prevent complications of aneurysm and occlusion. High-dose prednisolone, at 1 mg/kg (maximum of 60 mg), is advised for the first month and should then be gradually tapered. This improves constitutional symptoms and halts disease progression. Additional immunosuppressive agents should also be considered, particularly in those who fail to respond clinically initially or flare when the steroids are tapered. Preliminary small studies have shown benefit with the use of methotrexate, azathioprine, cyclophosphamide, mycophenolate mofetil, and infliximab. Other important management issues include hypertension and the prevention and treatment of thrombosis. Since TakA generally affects women of child-bearing age, management of hypertension in pregnancy is important.

TakA may result in permanent stenosis and the definitive treatment for occlusive disease is surgical. The indications for surgical treatment include:

- hypertension from coarctation of the aorta or renovascular disease
- end-organ or peripheral limb ischaemia
- arterial aneurysm or aortic regurgitation.

Surgical techniques include surgical bypass grafting, percutaneous transluminal angioplasty, and vascular stenting, and should be delayed until the acute phase is over to minimize the risk of procedural complications and re-occlusion.

4. Which imaging modalities may be useful in TakA?

A number of imaging modalities are useful for the investigation of patients presenting with symptoms suggestive of large-vessel vasculitis. These include conventional or digital subtraction angiography, MRI and MRA, CT and CT angiography, PET, and high-resolution ultrasound. Imaging is used to assess active inflammation in the vessel wall or structural changes. Conventional angiography has been the gold standard investigation of TakA, demonstrating vessel involvement such as luminal irregularity, stenosis, occlusion, and aneurysm formation. However, it does not provide information on arterial wall changes and exposes the patient to contrast media and radioactivity. Imaging with MRI/MRA avoids these risks and may demonstrate early vessel-wall thickening, typical of inflammatory lesions. It may be useful in disease monitoring. Ultrasound examination is also non-invasive and is increasingly used to assess large-vessel vasculitis. It is particularly useful for visualization of the common carotid and vertebral arteries but assessment of deeper vessels is limited. CT angiography with contrast enhancement demonstrates vessel wall oedema which may be associated with inflammation but has been shown to have poor correlation with progression of vascular lesions. It is also limited by the requirement of iodinated contrast and radiation exposure. FDG-PET demonstrates abnormal uptake of radioactive glucose in the wall for large vessels (>4 mm) and can detect pre-stenotic disease in patients presenting with non-specific features. It results in a significant radiation exposure and is an expensive procedure. It may be very useful in diagnosis but not as yet in assessment of disease activity or monitoring.

Further reading

Andrews J, Mason JC (2007). Takayasu's arteritis—recent advances in imaging offer promise. *Rheumatology*; **46**: 6–15.

Brunner J, Feldman BM, Tyrrell PN *et al.* (2010). Takayasu arteritis in children and adolescents. *Rheumatology*; **49**: 1806–14.

Johnston SL, Lock RJ, Gompels MM (2002). Takayasu arteritis: a review. *J Clin Pathol*; **55**: 481–6.

Maksimowicz-McKinnon K, Clark TM, Hoffman GS (2009). Takayasu arteritis and giant cell arteritis: a spectrum within the same disease? *Medicine*; **88**: 221–6.

Mukhtyar C, Guillevin L, Cid MC, *et al.* (2009). EULAR recommendations for the management of large vessel vasculitis. *Ann Rheum Dis*; **68**: 318–23.

Weyand CM, Goronzy J (2003). Medium and large vessel vasculitis. *N Eng J Med*; **349**: 160–9.

Case 41

A 27-year-old female with discoid lupus was referred to the rheumatology clinic with hand pain. Her pain was associated with episodic attacks of well-demarcated colour changes affecting both hands, usually on exposure to cold. She had not experienced any digital ulceration but was concerned that her lupus had become more systemic in nature. She smoked 20 cigarettes a day and drank eight cups of coffee a day. She had a past medical history of migraine and there was a family history of primary Raynaud's phenomenon in her aunt. She had recently been prescribed hydroxychloroquine and topical steroid therapy for a rash.

Examination of the rash revealed circular erythematous scaly lesions over her chest and proximal arms. Musculoskeletal examination was normal.

Investigations showed the following:

- Negative ANA
- Normal FBC, ESR, and complement levels
- Normal urinalysis.

Questions

1. What additional bedside test should be performed and what might it show?
2. Which conditions are associated with secondary Raynaud's phenomenon and how may the clinical presentation differ from primary Raynaud's?
3. What is known of the pathophysiology of Raynaud's phenomenon?
4. What are the treatment options for this condition?

Answers

1. What additional bedside test should be performed and what might it show?

Nailfold capilloroscopy enables the morphology of the capillaries to be examined in order to help distinguish between primary and secondary Raynaud's phenomenon. A drop of immersion oil is placed on the nailbed and the capillaries are examined using a magnifying lens. A normal appearance would show uniform morphology and homogenous distribution of the small capillary loops beneath the cuticle. In contrast, abnormal capillaroscopy findings show discrete dilated capillary loops and loss of surrounding loop structures. These findings are usually seen in the context of secondary Raynaud's phenomenon.

2. Which conditions are associated with a secondary Raynaud's phenomenon and how may the clinical presentation differ from primary Raynaud's?

Ten per cent of healthy people have primary or idiopathic Raynaud's phenomenon-which occurs in the absence of underlying disease. Secondary Raynaud's phenomenon (Raynaud's syndrome) is associated with an underlying disease. The distinguishing features are summarized in Table 41.1.

Table 41.1 Characteristics of primary and secondary Raynaud's phenomenon

Characteristic	Primary	Secondary
Age at onset	<30 years	>30 years
Associated autoimmune disease	No	Yes
Pattern of involvement	Symmetrical	Asymmetrical
Pain with attacks	Infrequent	Frequent
Trophic changes (digital ulceration, fissuring, gangrene)	Infrequent	More common
Nailfold capillaries	Normal	Abnormal
ESR	Normal	Elevated
Autoantibodies	Negative or low titres	Elevated titres

The conditions associated with secondary Raynaud's phenomenon include the following.

♦ Rheumatological disorders:
  • systemic sclerosis
  • systemic lupus erythematosus
  • dermatomyositis, polymyositis
  • Sjögren's syndrome
  • vasculitis.
♦ Traumatic:
  • vibration injury.

Other conditions that may mimic Raynaud's phenomenon are as follows.

♦ Vascular occlusive disease:
  • thromboembolic disease
  • arteriosclerosis
  • thoracic outlet syndrome.
♦ Drug-induced:
  • β-adrenergic blockers
  • cocaine
  • ciclosporin
  • vinblastine
  • bleomycin
  • cisplatin.
♦ Hyperviscosity disease:
  • polycythaemia
  • cryoglobulinaemia
  • paraproteinaemia.

Overall the features of this case are most consistent with a diagnosis of primary Raynaud's phenomenon. Although she has a diagnosis of cutaneous lupus, there is no evidence of any systemic complications and the lack of any associated trophic changes makes Raynaud's disease more likely. Furthermore, the family history and the past history of migraine and lifestyle habits put the patient at a higher risk of developing primary Raynaud's phenomenon.

3. What is known of the pathophysiology of Raynaud's phenomenon?

The exact pathophysiology is not fully understood, but the three main mechanisms can be divided into vascular, neural, and intravascular abnormalities.

In primary Raynaud's phenomenon the vascular abnormalities are likely to be functional compared to a combination of defective function and structure in secondary Raynaud's. Endothelial cells regulate vascular tone by producing a number of vasodilatory mediators, and a deficiency of nitric oxide (NO), one such vasodilator, has been implicated in the pathogenesis of Raynaud's. The contribution of vasoconstrictors such as endothelin-1 and angiotensin is also under investigation. The association of primary Raynaud's with migraine and Prinzmetal's angina suggests a systemic disorder rather than vasospasm isolated to the peripheries. Structural vascular changes seen in secondary Raynaud's include severe fibrotic proliferation of the intima with muscular hypertrophy. Such intimal pathology is often associated with intravascular thrombi, which can completely occlude the vessel lumen.

Neurotransmitters from autonomic and sensory afferent nerves alter digital vascular tone and are thought to be important in both primary and secondary disease. Neurotransmitters implicated include epinephrine, vasopressin, bradykinin, histamine, leukotrienes, and calcitonin gene-related peptide.

Several circulating factors have been implicated in the pathogenesis of Raynaud's phenomenon, especially in the context of systemic sclerosis. Platelet activation, defective fibrinolysis, and oxidant stress have all been implicated. The mechanisms are not fully understood, but it is thought that these intravascular factors may reduce basal blood flow in the microvasculature, in turn exacerbating the effect of digital vasospasm.

4. What are the treatment options for this condition?

The management of Raynaud's phenomenon depends on the severity of the disease, which can range from mild symptoms to digital ulceration and gangrene, and the presence of any underlying conditions. General treatment options are considered below.

Lifestyle modification

- Avoid exposure to sudden changes in ambient temperature
- Smoking cessation
- Avoid predisposing substances including caffeine.

Drug treatment

- **Calcium-channel blockers** have a vasodilatory effect with direct action on vascular smooth muscle, alongside inhibition of platelet activation. The dihydropyridine group (nifedipine, amlodipine, felodipine) is the least cardioselective and appears to be the most efficacious for the treatment of Raynaud's phenomenon. Adverse effects such as headaches and lower-extremity oedema result in discontinuation in many patients. Compliance can be enhanced by use of slow-release preparations and gradual dose escalation. Reflux symptoms can be exacerbated in patients with CREST as lower oesophageal sphincter tone is lowered. In patients with systemic sclerosis with moderate to severe pulmonary hypertension, vasodilator therapy should be introduced with caution as it can result in hypotension and associated vascular collapse.

- **Topical glyceryl trinitrate** has been shown to reduce the severity and number of attacks in both primary and secondary Raynaud's phenomenon. Frequent headaches often limit its use clinically.

- **Intravenous vasodilatory prostaglandins** are particularly effective in secondary Raynaud's phenomenon, improving both the Raynaud's attacks and digital ulceration. In addition to the affect on vascular tone, prostaglandins inhibit platelet aggregation. Iloprost, a prostaglandin analogue, may have additional antifibrotic activity. Common side effects include headache, hypotension, nausea, and flushing.

- **Phosphodiesterase inhibitors** such as sildenafil may be helpful in Raynaud's phenomenon by enhancing the vasodilatory effect of both nitrous oxide and prostaglandins. The evidence to date is inconclusive.

- **ACE inhibitors and angiotensin II receptor antagonists** are often used in the treatment of Raynaud's phenomenon, but the studies to date are inconclusive.

- **Endothelin receptor antagonists**, such as bosentan, are effective in the treatment of pulmonary hypertension and have been shown to improve healing of existing ulcers or improve Raynaud's attacks. Preliminary evidence suggests a role for the drug in the prevention of digital ulceration and amelioration of the symptoms from ulcers.

- **α-adrenergic receptor antagonists**, such as prazosin, show improvement in Raynaud's attacks but frequent side effects limit use. Newer agents are better tolerated and currently under investigation.

- **Anticoagulation and anti-thrombotic therapy** are often used in the context of severe digital ischaemia. Although the use of anti-thrombotic therapy is not evidence based, the use of low-dose daily aspirin in patients with severe ischaemia or ulceration is generally accepted. Anticoagulation is most effective in the context of an embolic or vascular occlusive process and is usually used as a short-term option. There is some pilot evidence for the use of longer-term heparin to reduce the severity of Raynaud's phenomenon, but the risk of adverse events necessitates more robust long-term evidence.

- **Ginkgo biloba** has also been shown to be effective in patients with Raynaud's disease.

Surgical treatment

Surgical treatment is usually reserved for patients with severe intractable digital ischaemia, which is most commonly seen in patients with underlying connective tissue disease.

- **Botulinum toxin** can be injected into affected digits and acts by eliminating presynaptic cholinergic inhibition of neurogenic relaxation. The consequent paralysis of digital artery muscle enhances digital blood flow. Botulinum toxin may also block stimulation of pain-transmitting C-fibres, ameliorating vasospasm-induced pain.

- **Chemical sympathectomy** is achieved by injecting anaesthetic near the appropriate cervical or lumbar sympathetic ganglia with temporary effect.
- **Cervical sympathectomy** is rarely recommended because of the associated complications such as Horner's syndrome and persistent neuralgia.
- **Surgical debridement** is the most common surgical technique employed in patients with Raynaud's phenomenon. Occasionally amputation is required for gangrene, intractable ulceration, or osteomyelitis.

Further reading

Bakst R, Merola JF, Franks AG Jr, Sanchez M (2008). Raynaud's phenomenon: pathogenesis and management. *J Am Acad Dermatol*; **59**: 633–53.

Lambova SN, Muller-Ladner U (2009). New lines in therapy of Raynaud's phenomenon. *Rheumatol Int*; **29**: 355–63.

Lambova SN, Muller-Ladner U (2009). The role of capillaroscopy in differentiation of primary and secondary Raynaud's phenomenon in rheumatic diseases: a review of the literature and two case reports. *Rheumatol Int*; **29**: 1263–71.

Case 42

A 10-year-old boy presented to his GP with a 4-week history of anterior chest wall pain exacerbated by deep inspiration that was severe enough to prevent him attending school. On examination he was systemically well, but had tenderness over the sternum and right second rib, which appeared prominent. A CXR showed a lytic lesion of the right second rib (Fig. 42.1). He was referred to the orthopaedic team. Given the uncertain nature of the lesion it was thought prudent to commence treatment for osteomyelitis with intravenous antibiotics. Blood cultures taken prior to treatment were subsequently found to be negative.

Investigations showed the following:

- Hb 10.4 g/dL; WCC 11.5 × 10⁹/L; platelets 552 × 10⁹/L; MCV 76.8 fL
- ESR 62 mm/h; CRP 48.2 mg/L
- CXR—see Fig. 42.1 for image of upper chest
- MRI scan—see Figs 42.2 and 42.3
- Bone biopsy: mixed acute and chronic inflammatory cell infiltrate in the marrow spaces with numerous polymorphs extending into the surrounding soft tissue and muscle in keeping with infection. No organisms seen on Gram staining.

Osteomyelitis was considered the most likely initial diagnosis and he underwent a 6-week course of empirical intravenous ceftriaxone followed by a 6-month course of doxycycline and rifampicin. At his annual review he was pain free and a follow-up MRI scan demonstrated partial resolution of the rib and sternal lesions.

However, he presented again at the age of 13 years with pain in the same rib and upper chest wall, right hip, and lower back. During the subsequent year, he developed a pustular skin eruption on his finger and joint pain and swelling of his wrists, fingers, and knees. He underwent a technetium bone scan (Fig. 42.4).

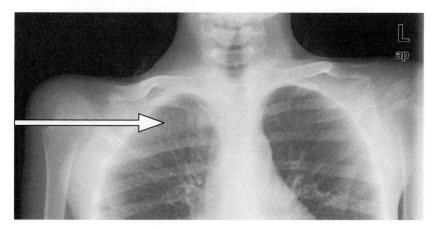

Fig. 42.1 X-ray of the upper chest. The arrow shows the site of the lytic lesion.

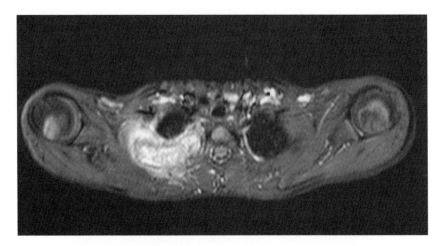

Fig. 42.2 MRI scan of the chest.

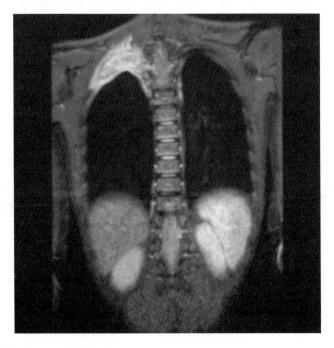

Fig. 42.3 MRI scan of the chest.

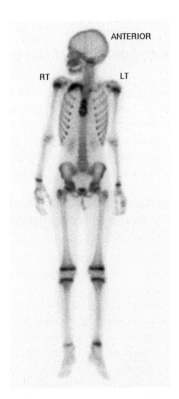

Fig. 42.4 Technetium bone scan.

Questions

1. What is demonstrated on the MRI and technetium bone scans?
2. What are the important differential diagnoses, and what was the most likely cause of his symptoms?
3. What is the rash likely to be?
4. How would you manage this case?

Answers

1. What is demonstrated on the MRI and technetium bone scans?

The X-ray of the upper chest (Fig. 42.1) shows an osteolytic lesion of the right second rib. The MRI scans (Figs 42.2 and 42.3) show expansion and destruction of the right second rib with involvement of the sternum. An abnormal signal suggesting oedema can be seen to extend into the surrounding soft tissues. The technetium bone scan (Fig. 42.4) demonstrates multiple areas of increased uptake, in particular right hip, left ankle, sternum, and upper two right ribs.

2. What are the important differential diagnoses, and what was the most likely cause of his symptoms?

The two most important differentials at presentation were infection and malignancy. His initial presentation with pain, a lytic lesion on X-ray, and histological features of chronic inflammation was in keeping with infection although no organism was identified.

Children with bone tumours may present with pain, which is often worse at night, localized tenderness, and swelling. Systemic features are absent in patients with benign lesions, but fever and weight loss may occur with malignancies. Benign tumours include osteoid osteoma and osteoblastoma (an osteoid osteoma >2 cm in diameter), which both occur more frequently in boys. Eosinophilic granuloma is a localized Langerhans cell histiocytosis, characteristically occurring in children between 5 and 10 years of age and is seen as a lytic lesion on X-ray. Malignant musculoskeletal tumours of childhood include osteogenic sarcoma, rhabdomyosarcoma, and Ewing's sarcoma.

This child presented over 3 years with a number of inflammatory bone lesions but was systemically well. There was partial resolution of the initial lesion followed by the development of inflammatory bone lesions at other sites and new skin and joint disease. Although histological examination of the lesions demonstrated features typical of infection, no organism was identified and the response to antibiotics was variable. The clinical picture evolved to include a pustular skin rash and joint inflammation. The bone lesions are typical of chronic relapsing multifocal osteomyelitis (CRMO) with progression of the disease to the SAPHO syndrome (synovitis, acne, pustulosis, hyperostosis, and osteitis).

CRMO and SAPHO form part of the same syndrome and have identical bone pathology, with CRMO occurring more commonly in children. CRMO is at the more severe end of a spectrum of inflammatory bone lesions termed chronic non-bacterial osteomyelitis. Histologically the lesions are identical to bacterial osteomyelitis but are not associated with infection. Lesions may occur at any skeletal site, but predominantly affect the metaphyses of long bones in children. It generally occurs at a median age of 10 years and is twice as frequent in females as in males.

CRMO has been associated with the spondyloarthropathies and may form part of enthesitis-related arthritis in children. However, the frequency of HLA B27 is the same as in the general population. An association with IBD has also been reported.

The SAPHO syndrome includes the same inflammatory bone lesions together with skin and joint manifestations. The clinical features of the SAPHO syndrome may not all be present at the outset; in particular, skin involvement may be absent. It may initially present in children and adults as CRMO alone, as in this case. A slight to moderate increase in inflammatory markers is common and there are no associated autoantibodies. Diagnosis is based on clinical, radiological, and histological findings.

A patient with SAPHO usually has multiple bony lesions affecting the anterior chest wall, rib cage, spine, metaphyses of lamellar bone, pelvis, and mandible. There may be a soft tissue component, as in this patient. The anterior chest wall, involving the sternoclavicular joint, is the most common site affected in 65–90% of patients. The spine is affected in 33% of patients and often involves the thoracic spine in the form of spondylodiscitis, osteosclerosis, and paravertebral ossifications. The sacroiliac joint may be involved. Long bones are involved in 30% of patients and flat bones, including the mandible and ilium, in 10% of patients. Solitary bone lesions may occur and are most often present in the clavicle or mandible. Peripheral arthritis has been reported in 92% of cases of SAPHO.

The most prominent feature on X-ray is the presence of hyperostosis and osteitis. CT and MRI are useful for localizing lesions. Appearances can be similar to that of chronic osteomyelitis but there is no sequestrum or abscess formation. MRI is also useful in follow-up where T_2-weighted sequences with fat suppression identify bone marrow oedema. Technetium bone scans can identify clinically silent lesions. Imaging does not exclude malignancy, particularly in unifocal lesions where biopsy needs to be considered.

The diagnostic criteria for SAPHO put forward by Kahn and colleagues in 1994 are as follows.

♦ Chronic relapsing multifocal osteomyelitis involving the axial or peripheral skeleton:
  • usually sterile or with the presence of *Propionbacterium acnes*
  • spine may be involved
  • with or without skin lesions.

♦ Acute, subacute, or chronic arthritis with any of the following:
  • palmoplantar pustulosis
  • pustular psoriasis
  • severe acne/hydradenitis.

♦ Any severe osteitis with any of following:
  • palmoplantar pustulosis
  • pustular psoriasis
  • severe acne or hydradenitis.

Any one of the three presentations is sufficient for diagnosis.

3. What is the rash likely to be?

The pustular skin eruption on his finger is likely to be a palmoplantar pustulosis which is the most common skin manifestation associated with SAPHO and is thought to represent a variation of psoriasis vulgaris. The prevalence of psoriasis in SAPHO is three times that in the general population.

Dermatological manifestations of SAPHO are generally neutrophilic pustular disorders:

- psoriasis (pustular psoriasis, palmar-plantar pustulosis)
- acne (acne conglobata, acne fulminans, or follicular occlusion triad).

Other associated skin diseases include hydradenitis suppurativa, pyoderma gangrenosum, dissecting scalp cellulitis, and Sweet's syndrome, all of which are pseudo-abscesses.

4. How would you manage this case?

Initial management of inflammatory bone pain should be with an NSAID such as ibuprofen 30 mg/kg/day or naproxen 15–20 mg/kg/day and is effective in 80% of cases. Bisphosphonates are potent inhibitors of osteoclastic activity, and the nitrogen-containing bisphosphonate pamidronate has anti-inflammatory and pain-modifying activity.

There are reports of successful treatment with corticosteroids and DMARDs, and these may be useful in controlling inflammatory joint disease. There are case reports of a partial response to biological therapies such as infliximab and adalimumab in children with CRMO but not with anakinra. Severe skin lesions may respond to topical steroid creams.

This boy was treated with NSAIDs, but continued to experience bone pain which responded well to a course of pamidronate infusions. His joint and skin disease was successfully treated with methotrexate 15 mg/m². He had become deconditioned because of poor mobility during prolonged periods of pain, and required support from physiotherapy and occupational therapy in order to return to full activities.

Further reading

Catalano-Pons C, Comte A, Wipff J, et al. (2008). Clinical outcome in children with CRMO. Rheumatology 47: 1397–9.

Eleftheriou D, Gerschman T, Sebire N, Woo P, Pilkington CA, Brogan PA (2010). Biological therapy in refractory chronic non-bacterial osteomyelitis of childhood. Rheumatology; 49: 1505–12.

Girschick HJ, Raab P, Surbaum S, et al. (2005). Chronic non-bacterial osteomyelitis in children Ann Rheum Dis; 64: 279–85.

Huber AM, Lam PY, Duffy CM, et al. (2002). CRMO: clinical outcomes after more than five years of follow-up. J Paediatr; 141: 198–203.

Jansson A, Renner ED, Ramser J, et al. (2007). Classification of non-bacterial osteitis. Retrospective study of clinical immunological and genetic aspects in 89 patients. Rheumatology; 46; 154–60.

Job-Deslandre C, Krebs S, Kahan A (2001). Chronic recurrent multifocal osteomyelitis: five-year outcomes in 14 paediatric cases. *Joint Bone Spine*; **68**: 245–51.

Kahn MF, Khan MA (1994), The SAPHO syndrome. *Baillière's Clin Rheumatol*; **8**: 333–62.

Kahn MF (1993). Psoriatic arthritis and synovitis, acne, pustulosis, hyperostosis, and osteitis syndrome. *Curr Opin Rheumatol*; **5**: 428–35.

Kerrison C, Davidson JE, Cleary AG, Beresford MW (2004). Pamidronate in the treatment of childhood SAPHO syndrome. *Rheumatology*; **43**: 1246–51.

Vittecoq O, Said LA, Michot C, *et al.* (2000). Evolution of chronic recurrent multifocal osteomyelitis toward spondylarthropathy over the long term. *Arthritis Rheum*; **43**: 109–19.

Case 43

An 18-year-old nursery nurse presented with a 6-week history of a painful migratory arthritis affecting her right ankle, left knee, and right wrist. She had a pale pink non-irritant rash on both forearms at the onset of illness which settled after a week.

As a child she had missed schooling because of recurrent tonsillitis. At age 11 years she had been diagnosed with an irritable hip which had resolved spontaneously. She lived with her parents and worked full time in a crèche looking after preschool children. She had returned from a camping holiday in Brittany 6 weeks before the onset of arthritis. She remembered no insect bites and had no regular sexual partner. Her paternal grandmother had rheumatic fever in childhood.

On examination she was afebrile, had normal skin and nails, blood pressure 90/60 mmHg, a regular pulse of 80 beats/min, and a grade 2/6 basal systolic murmur. Her right wrist was swollen and very tender but had a full range of passive movement. The overlying skin was warm and erythematous. Her other joints and spine were normal.

Investigations showed the following:

◆ Hb 12.3 g/dL; WCC 7.4×10^9/L; platelets 486×10^9/L

◆ CRP 72 mg/L

◆ CXR normal

◆ ECG normal.

Questions

1. What is the differential diagnosis?
2. What further history and investigations will aid diagnosis?
3. What treatment options are available?

Answers

1. What is the differential diagnosis?

- Viral related arthritis
- Reactive arthritis
- Post-streptococcal reactive arthritis
- Acute rheumatic fever
- Other infection-related arthritis (e.g. Lyme disease, *Brucella*, *Gonococcus*)
- Early inflammatory arthritis
- Connective tissue disease.

This patient is at risk of viral-related arthritis as her employment brings her into contact with young children. The personal and family history of tonsillitis and rheumatic fever raises the possibility of post-streptococcal-related arthritis or atypical rheumatic fever. The recent camping holiday in France raise the possibilities of reactive arthritis, gonococcal arthritis, Lyme disease, and brucellosis. Early inflammatory arthritis and SLE can present with migratory arthritis symptoms. The systolic murmur may be functional, long-standing, or part of the acute illness and needs investigation.

2. What further history and investigations will aid diagnosis?

Viral-related arthritis

Viral-related arthritis is common in children and young adults. The most common presentation is a symmetrical peripheral arthritis. Transient rashes are common and non-specific. Most are benign and resolve within 6 weeks, and patients only present if the problem is severe or persistent. Rheumatoid factor and ANA may be transiently positive during the acute phase. Diagnostic signs and symptoms of specific viral illnesses may develop after the arthritis and rash have resolved.

- Parvovirus B19 is common, with presentations differing between children and adults. Seventy per cent of children are asymptomatic, but some have mild flu-like symptoms and a bright red rash ('slapped cheek'); joint symptoms are rare. In adults the rash is rare and joint symptoms occur in up to 60% with arthralgia or a symmetrical peripheral small-joint arthritis resembling early rheumatoid arthritis. This resolves almost universally within 3 months. Some adults have a transient aplastic crisis, particularly those with hereditary spherocytosis. Maternal infection during pregnancy can lead to fetal hydramnios and first- and second-trimester abortion.
- EBV infection is common in older teenagers and can be associated with polyarthralgia, polyarthritis, or a self-limiting monoarthritis.
- Adenovirus and Coxsackie virus infections can be associated with rashes, polyarthritis, pleurisy, pericarditis, or myocarditis.

- Mumps in adults can present with small- or large-joint arthritis which takes several weeks to settle and can occur up to 4 weeks before the parotitis develops.
- Adult rubella can present with peripheral polyarthritis and morning stiffness before the rash appears. Arthritis associated with rubella and mumps is rare in the UK because of the successful vaccination programme.
- Hepatitis B presents with symmetrical large-joint and hand arthritis which may be migratory or persistent. Arthritis and an associated urticaria may precede the jaundice by weeks and persist after the acute hepatitis has settled. Transmission is by blood products or sexual contact.
- HIV-related arthritis can be highly variable, ranging from mild arthralgia to debilitating arthritis which is usually monoarticular.

Reactive arthritis

It is important to exclude reactive arthritis. The arthritis is often mono- or oligoarticular and persistent, but can be migratory. A careful history about risk of gastrointestinal or genitourinary infections is needed. Genitourinary infections in particular may be silent in females, or patients may not volunteer symptoms because of embarrassment or lack of understanding of any connection with arthritis symptoms. Associated skin rashes include palmar pustulosis, keratoderma blenhorragica, and erythema nodosum. Rarely, aortic valve disease and conduction abnormalities can occur.

Streptococcal-related arthritis

It is important to consider a diagnosis of acute rheumatic fever or post-streptococcal-related arthritis, as cardiac involvement occurs with recurrent episodes and can be prevented by prophylactic penicillin. Rheumatic fever typically affects preschool children but can occur in older children and young adults, particularly in an institutional setting. In rheumatic fever, the arthritis is migratory and the joints involved are often exquisitely tender, disproportionate to the physical signs. The arthritis and synovitis usually resolve spontaneously within a week. Post-streptococcal-related arthritis is usually a more persistent large-joint oligoarticular arthritis. Cardiac involvement is less common but late cardiac complications have occurred in 10% of patients.

The diagnosis of acute rheumatic fever was modified in 1992 to include major criteria of carditis, polyarthritis, erythema marginatum, subcutaneous nodules, and chorea. Minor criteria are a prolonged PR interval on ECG, arthralgia, fevers, and raised acute phase response. One major and two minor criteria are needed with evidence of antecedent streptococcal infection from throat swab culture or serial bloods for antistreptococcal antibodies.

Skin involvement includes the characteristic evanescent erythema marginatum which is pink or red, resolves from the centre, and is associated with carditis. Painless firm subcutaneous nodules may mimic rheumatoid arthritis.

Pericarditis can affect any part of the heart including conduction defects in heart block, valvular lesions affecting the aortic and mitral valve, pericarditis, and heart failure.

Neurological sequelae include chorea (involuntary purposeless movements, grimaces of hands and face), muscular weakness, and emotional changes ranging from irritability to psychosis.

Both post-streptococcal-reactive arthritis and acute rheumatic fever forms are non-suppurative sequelae of group A β-haemolytic streptococcal infection. The other important condition is acute glomerulonephritis. Different M serotypes of the group A streptococci are associated with these different sequelae (nephritogenic, arthritogenic, and cardiogenic). There has been a recent resurgence in post-streptococcal-related illness which may be related to change in virulence and prevalence of different M serotypes.

Host factors affecting susceptibility may include age, gender, associated viral infections, and genetic background. Acute rheumatic fever is more common in first-degree relatives of patients.

Lyme disease

Lyme disease is increasing in prevalence, particularly in southwest Britain during late spring and summer. The infective organism *Borrelia* is a Gram-negative spirochete transmitted via tick bites. Three species are found in Europe (*Borrelia burgdorferi*, *Borrelia garnii*, and *Borrelia afzelii*) and each presents with different clinical manifestations, although all three can cause arthritis. The pathognomonic rash of erythema chronicum migrans occurs within a few days to a month after the bite. It is classically a purple-red well-demarcated rash near the site of the tick bite which can take up to 4 weeks to settle. Patients often do not recall a tick bite. Lymphadenopathy, conjunctivitis, and systemic malaise can follow. Joint pains are often migratory but a chronic arthritis, commonly affecting the knee, can develop. Fifty-five per cent develop carditis with conduction problems. Acute neuroborreliosis occurs in 10–15% of patients, presenting as meningitis, facial nerve palsy, which is often bilateral (or other cranial neuropathies), painful sensorimotor, or radiculopathy. Diagnosis of early Lyme disease is by detection of a rise in IgM antibodies which peak 6–8 weeks after exposure.

Gonococcal infection

Gonococcal infection (see Case 37) can cause both septic and reactive arthritis and is often associated with tenosynovitis. Patients are usually febrile and may present with asymmetrical migratory polyarthralgia. The associated papular or vesicular non-itchy rash occurs on trunk and limbs, with facial sparing. Joint aspiration is needed to distinguish between septic arthritis and reactive arthritis. Pancarditis including conduction disturbance can occur, as can osteomyelitis, hepatitis, and meningitis.

Brucellosis

Unpasteurized cheese is widely eaten in France and may be a source of brucellosis in the current case. Septic arthritis is a common complication of *Brucella* infection, presenting as a large-joint monoarthritis or unilateral sacroiliitis or spondylitis. Transient reactive symmetrical peripheral polyarthritis can also occur. Endocarditis occurs infrequently, usually affects the aortic valve, and is a life-threatening complication.

Blood tests show anaemia, leucopenia, and sometimes thrombocytopenia with an inflammatory response. Joint aspiration is usually sterile. Prolonged culture (6 weeks) of the organism from blood and bone marrow is the current gold standard for diagnosis. A new PCR assay has been developed which can provide positive results in 10 days.

Connective tissue disease and early inflammatory arthritis

Connective tissue disease and early inflammatory arthritis should be considered. SLE is more common in young women who may present with rash, arthritis, and carditis (see case 9). ANA is a useful screening test but may be transiently raised during any acute infection.

Early rheumatoid arthritis can present as palindromic rheumatism with a migratory, often large-joint, arthritis. Joint symptoms flare to a peak and resolve completely in hours or days. Patients are well between attacks. Up to one-third of patients subsequently go on to develop persistent rheumatoid arthritis.

Psoriatic and enteropathic arthritis may present with a short-lived migratory arthritis. Psoriatic rashes may be short-lived and a family history is important, particularly in the young.

Further investigations

- Throat swabs for β-haemolytic streptococcus are positive in a third of patients without prior antibiotics, and in a tenth with prior antibiotics. Serial blood samples for streptococcal serology such as ASOT and anti-DNAse B: single tests give 80% sensitivity; two tests increase sensitivity to 90%.
- RF and ANA may both be transiently raised during acute infections and settle to normal. The test should be interpreted in the clinical context.
- Viral serology to demonstrate a rise in serial IgM antibody titres during an acute illness, or a slower rise in IgG titres after the acute illness.
- Hepatitis B serology and HIV status if appropriate.
- Stool sample: most commont organisms associated with reactive arthritis are *Campylobacter*, *Salmonella*, *Shigella*, and *Yersinia*.
- Genitourinary investigation for *Chlamydia*, *Gonococcus*, and syphilis.
- ECG to look for conduction abnormalities, PR interval, and tachycardia.
- CXR.
- Echocardiogram to look for structural valvular lesions or pericardial effusion.

3. What treatment options are available?

- Most viral-related arthritis is self-limiting, as are most cases of reactive arthritis. NSAIDs and analgesics are helpful in symptom relief.

- Intra-articular corticosteroid injections can help resolve the joint swelling of reactive arthritis. This may be important to help patients return to work.
- Antibiotic treatment of the underlying infection in reactive arthritis is an independent consideration and does not speed arthritis resolution.
- Reactive arthritis patients who are HLA B27 positive are at increased risk of developing a persistent oligoarthritis or even spondylarthritis. These patients usually respond to a prolonged course of DMARDs such as sulfasalazine, methotrexate, or leflunomide.
- Early-stage Lyme disease with arthritis is treated with doxycycline plus amoxicillin for 30 days.
- Brucellosis requires prolonged combination antibiotic therapy for 6 weeks to 3 months.

This patient's throat swab grew β-haemolytic streptococcus and her sequential serological testing showed a rise in both ASOT and anti-DNAseB titres. ECG, CXR, and echocardiogram showed structurally normal heart valves with a rim of pericardial fluid. This was shown to resolve over the following 3 weeks. The systolic murmur was thought to be physiological. The diagnosis was of acute rheumatic fever.

The childhood episode of irritable hip may have been a previous attack of rheumatic fever. The transient rash may have been erythema multiforme. Although rheumatic fever usually occurs in childhood, 15% of first attacks occur in adults. The risk of carditis is >30% in the first attacks and increases with subsequent attacks. Treatment is 2–4 weeks of full-dose oral penicillin followed by long-term low-dose penicillin prophylaxis to prevent recurrent attacks with subsequent carditis.

The duration of penicillin prophylaxis depends on the risk of future group A streptococcal infection. In her case this would for as long as she was in contact with small children, which may be up to 10 years or even lifelong. Some consider post-streptococcal reactive arthritis a forme fruste of rheumatic fever, and even though the carditis risk is lower they advocate similar penicillin prophylaxis regimes.

Further reading

Bardin T (2003). Gonoccocal arthritis. *Best Pract Res Clin Rheumatol*; **17**: 201–8.

Cilliers AM (2006). Rheumatic fever and its management. *BMJ*; **337**: 1153–6.

Jansen T, Janssen M, van Reil P (1998). Acute rheumatic fever or post-streptococcal reactive arthritis: a clinical problem revisited. *Br J Rheumatol*; **37**: 335–40.

Medina Rodriguez F (2003). Rheumatic manifestations of human immunodeficiency virus *Rheum Dis Clin North Am*; **29**: 145–61.

Moore T (2000). Parvovirus-associated arthritis. *Curr Opin Rheumatol*; **12**: 289–94.

Pappas G, Akritidis N, Bosilkovski M, Tsianos E (2005). Brucellosis. *N Engl J Med*; **352**: 2325–36.

Schnarr S, Franz J, Krause A, Zeidler H (2006). Lyme borreliosis. *Best Pract Res Clin Rheumatol*; **20**: 1099–1118.

Case 44

A 55-year-old woman presented with a 5-year history of pain and swelling in her hands and feet with bilateral numbness and tingling in the median nerve distribution. She had gained 10 kg in weight over the same period of time and developed type 2 diabetes. She attributed increasing fatigue to poor sleep quality because of backache and to snoring.

On examination, she weighed 80 kg with a BMI of 35.2 kg/m². Her BP was 150/100 mmHg. She had a kyphosis and painful spinal movements. She had hand joint tenderness with generalized hand swelling and coarse thickened skin. Her wrists, knees, and ankles were hypermobile.

Investigations showed the following:

- Normal FBC and inflammatory markers
- R12 IU/ml; ACCP <6 U/ml
- Na 136 mmol/L; K 4.2 mmol/L; creatinine 70 μmol/L; total calcium 2.7 mmol/L; phosphate 1.04 mmol/L; ALT 30 IU/L; ALP 68 IU/L; albumin 40 g/L
- TSH 3.8 mU/L; PTH 60 ng/L
- Hand X-rays are shown in Fig. 44.1.

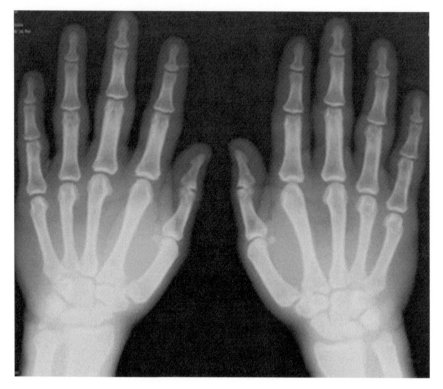

Fig. 44.1 X-ray of the patient's hands.

Questions

1. What metabolic diseases cause arthropathy?
2. What is the most likely diagnosis?
3. What do the hand X-rays show? What other imaging would be useful?
4. What is characteristic about this arthropathy and how should it be managed in the short and long term?

Answers

1. What metabolic diseases cause arthropathy?

Metabolic causes of arthropathy include:

- hypothyroidism
- hyperthyroidism
- diabetes
- diffuse idiopathic skeletal hyperostosis (DISH syndrome)
- primary hyperlipidaemias
- haemochromatosis
- acromegaly.

Hypothyroidism should be considered in all patients with carpal tunnel syndrome. It may occur in up to 10% of cases and is due to peripheral tissue oedema in the wrist. It would also account for the patient's weight gain, fatigue, and skin changes. Thyroid acropachy is a skeletal abnormality specific to Graves' disease; it is a painless swelling of the fingers and toes which may be associated with clubbing and periostitis.

Diabetics may develop a number of joint-related problems. Diabetic cheiroarthropathy is most common in type 1 disease, but may occur in type 2 diabetes. Patients develop soft tissue contractures that limit extension of the metacarpophalangeal (MCP) and interphalangeal (IP) joints without evidence of intra-articular or muscle inflammation. Patients with diabetic osteo-arthropathy develop destructive lytic joint lesions in association with peripheral neuropathy in type 2 diabetes. Hyperostotic spondylosis or DISH syndrome are more common in, although not confined to type 2 diabetics.

DISH is caused by widespread new bone formation with general ossification of ligaments and tendons, especially the anterior longitudinal ligament of the spine. It is most characteristic in the thoracic spine, but may cause stiffening and arthropathy in peripheral joints with reduced flexion of the fingers. Its association with the metabolic syndrome is thought to be related to hyperinsulinaemia and disturbances of GH.

Primary hyperlipidaemias are rarely associated with arthritis. Tendinous xanthomas are a recognized feature of some forms of familial hypercholesterolaemias.

Haemochromatosis is an inherited disease where increased iron absorption results in iron loading of tissues. It presents with fatigue and a symmetrical arthropathy in middle-aged patients. Liver abnormalities are demonstrated by chronic ALT elevation and type 2 diabetes may occur. It characteristically causes osteoarthritis of the second and third MCP joints, but can affect other joints.

2. What is the most likely diagnosis?

The most likely diagnosis is acromegaly. This patient had developed arthralgia with bilateral carpal tunnel syndrome, weight gain, diabetes, and hypertension. She had normal TFTs. She was hypercalcaemic with a normal PTH. The diagnosis of acromegaly was confirmed by a raised insulin-like growth factor 1 (IGF-1) of 78.4 nmol/L and failure of GH to suppress during a glucose tolerance test.

Acromegaly is caused by the hypersecretion of GH from a pituitary adenoma resulting in elevated IGF-I. Both hormones contribute to the features of the disease. It is rare with a prevalence of 50–70 cases per million and an incidence of 3–4 new cases per million per year. Characteristic changes caused by tissue overgrowth include coarsened facial features, exaggerated growth of hands and feet, soft tissue hypertrophy, and macroglossia. Thickening of the skin is a manifestation of the effect of GH on collagen tissue. There is softening and thickening of the capsular and ligamentous structures, resulting in joint laxity. Metabolic consequences include increased insulin resistance and hypercalcaemia. Poor-quality sleep and snoring are commonly reported. Increased mortality is due to cardiovascular, cerebrovascular, and respiratory disease.

3. What do the hand X-rays show? What other imaging would be useful?

The X-rays of the patient's hands (Fig. 44.1) show soft tissue thickening, increased joint space, and enlargement and tufting of the terminal phalanges. An MRI of her pituitary fossa demonstrated a pituitary adenoma. Heel-pad thickening, demonstrated on a lateral radiograph, is also a confirmatory sign.

Joint-space widening is most frequently observed in the knees and in the MCP and IP joints. The epiphyses may undergo squaring and develop small osteophytes on the edges of the articular surfaces, especially in the MCP joints. Acromegaly is characterized by new bone formation and by subcutaneous soft tissue and cartilage thickening. Axial arthropathy is a common finding and may affect the whole spine. Imaging of the spine demonstrates widened intervertebral spaces, vertebral enlargement, and osteophyte formation with calcification of the intervertebral ligaments, resembling the changes observed in DISH.

4. What is characteristic about this arthropathy and how should it be managed in the short and long term?

Arthropathy is a well-established feature of acromegaly and may be the first presentation of the disease. Joint symptoms or signs occur in 60–70% patients. Acromegalic arthropathy has a characteristic biphasic presentation. In the first phase, soft tissue and cartilage hypertrophy result in joint widening and hypermobility. Chronic secretion of GH stimulates production of both circulating and local cartilage IGF-I. This induces chondrocyte proliferation and cartilage matrix synthesis, with cartilage thickening which can be demonstrated by ultrasound. GH causes growth of fibroblasts and collagen formation with enlargement of ligaments and joint laxity. Bilateral carpal tunnel syndrome frequently occurs and is caused by both compression and hypertrophy of the median nerve.

With time the thickened poor-quality cartilage wears unevenly and fissures form, leading to exposure of subchondral bone. Joint stability is compromised by ligament laxity and synovial hypertrophy with effusions. Secondary osteoarthritic changes affect both axial and peripheral joints, especially weight-bearing joints, and may be severe.

The initial treatment of acromegaly is with trans-sphenoidal surgery to remove the pituitary tumour. Radiotherapy and medical treatment with somatostatin analogues, such as octreotide (a long-acting analogue of somatostatin), or pegvisomant (a GH antagonist) may be required. Reversal of cartilage widening has been demonstrated with ultrasound. Surgical carpal tunnel decompression may be required. Although the first stage of acromegalic arthropathy may be reversible, secondary osteoarthritis changes may cause severe joint disease affecting both the axial and the appendicular skeleton. This should be managed with analgesia, physiotherapy, occupational therapy, and orthotics before consideration of joint replacement. The use of NSAIDs is relatively contraindicated in view of the increased risk of cardiovascular disease; 35% patients with acromegaly develop hypertension.

Borderline or raised serum calcium may occur in acromegaly and is attributed to vitamin D activation by GH independent of PTH. However, the most common reason for hypercalcaemia in acromegaly, occurring in 5–10% of patients, is a parathyroid-secreting adenoma and is associated with multiple endocrine neoplasia I (MEN-I) syndrome.

Further reading

Colao A, Cannavo S, Marzullo P, *et al.* (2003). Twelve months of treatment with octreotide-LAR reduces joint thickness in acromegaly. *Eur J Endocrinol*; **148**: 31–8.

Wassenaar MJE, Biermasz NR, van Duinen N, *et al.* (2009). High prevalence of arthropathy, according to the definitions of radiological and clinical osteoarthritis in patients with long-term cure of acromegaly: a case–control study. *Eur J Endocrinol*; **160**: 357–65.

Case 45

A 45-year-old woman with a 2-year history of increasing unsteadiness was referred from neurology to the rheumatology department. She had a 10-year history of chronic fatigue, arthralgia, and myalgia. She had a history of photosensitive rash. She had stopped wearing contact lenses in her early twenties because of symptomatic dry eyes, carried a water bottle with her to work, and had a constant irritating dry cough. She had two healthy children. One baby had had a transient neonatal rash. Her sister had autoimmune thyroid disease.

On examination, she was obese and normotensive, with tender but not swollen wrist, finger, and knee joints. She had significant dental caries. She had a wide-based staggering gait and was unable to heel–toe walk. Neurological examination was otherwise normal.

Investigations showed the following:

- Hb 12.4 g/L; WCC 3.8×10^9/L; lymphocyte 0.87×10^9/L
- Liver and renal function were normal
- RF negative; ANA 1 in 80
- Visual evoked responses were normal
- Lumbar puncture for oligoclonal bands were matched in CSF and serum
- MRI scan of brain showed extensive periventricular white matter changes in the frontal, parietal and occipital lobes (Fig. 45.1).

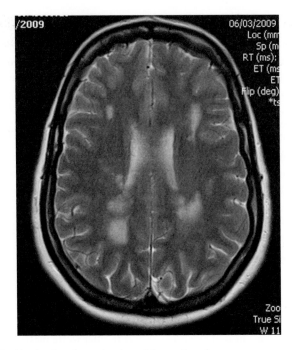

Fig. 45.1 MRI of brain showing extensive white matter changes.

Questions

1. This patient presents with a rare complication of a common connective tissue problem. What is the underlying diagnosis?

2. What bedside tests, blood tests, and laboratory tests will help to confirm the diagnosis of the connective tissue disease?

3. What are the common presentations of this condition and the treatment options?

4. What possible late complications occur?

Answers

1. This patient presents with a rare complication of a common connective tissue problem. What is the underlying diagnosis?

The diagnosis is primary Sjögren's syndrome (pSS) with Sjögren's myelopathy.

Neurological Sjögren's syndrome occurs in 1–5% of pSS patients. Clinical presentation is highly variable and can affect the peripheral and central nervous systems, cognitive function, and psychological state. Reported presentations include sensorimotor peripheral neuropathy, mononeuritis multiplex, optic neuropathy, cognitive dysfunction, and acute and chronic transverse myelitis. Neurological symptoms precede diagnosis of pSS in 81% of patients.

2. What bedside tests, blood tests, and laboratory tests will help to confirm the diagnosis of the connective tissue disease?

- Schirmer's test for tear-flow: a simple bedside testing using blotting paper strips to measure tear-flow over a 5 min period (positive test ≤5 mm in 5 min).
- Immunology tests for anti-Ro or anti-La antibodies or both. In most published series autoimmune serology for anti-Ro and anti-La antibodies is positive in 60% of pSS patients.
- Histopathology—minor salivary gland biopsy (Fig. 45.2).

CNS lesions can be very difficult to distinguish from multiple sclerosis (MS) on MRI. MRI lesions of pSS resemble multiple-sclerosis-like deposits, but are more diffuse. Clinically, it can also be difficult to distinguish CSF in Sjögren's syndrome from that in multiple sclerosis, and the visual evoked potential responses can be

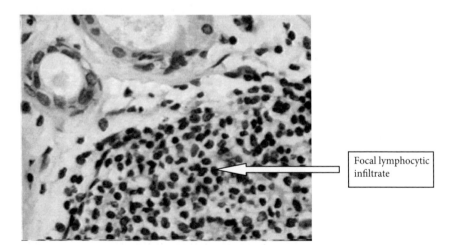

Focal lymphocytic infiltrate

Fig. 45.2 (See also Plate 17) Histology of the minor salivary gland.

positive in both. The main distinguishing feature is that matched oligoclonal bands are present in both CSF and blood, whereas in multiple sclerosis they are present only in the CSF.

The American–European Consensus Group (AECG) classification criteria for pSS require four out of six positive, including either histopathology or serology.

- Ocular symptoms—persistent troublesome dry eyes daily for more than 3 months, or current sensation of sand or gravel in the eyes or need for tear substitute more than three times daily.

- Oral symptoms—daily feeling of dry mouth for >3 months, or current persistently swollen salivary glands in adults, or frequently drinking liquids to aid swallowing dry food.

- Objective dry eyes—positive Schirmer's Test (≤5 mm in 5 min) or positive Rose Bengal score.

- Histopathology—minor salivary gland biopsy showing focal lymphocytic sialadenitis, ductal hyperplasia, and acinar atrophy.

- A positive biopsy has, on focus, >50 lymphocytes per 4 mm^2 tissue. The predominant lymphocyte is type CD4 positive.

- Objective dry mouth: unstimulated whole salivary flow <1.5 mL/15 min or parotid sialography showing diffuse sialectasis without major duct involvement or salivary scintigraphy showing delayed uptake of tracer.

- Serology: positive Ro or positive La antibodies or both.

3. What are the common presentations of this condition and the treatment options?

Patients with Sjögren's syndrome often present late, in part because they adapt to the symptoms and also because there is significant salivary and tear reserve. The salivary flow rate may fall as low as 30–40% of normal before patients complain of dry mouth. Although dry eyes and dry mouth are the most common presenting features, patients often present to general practice or other specialities. Common symptoms include fatigue, arthralgia, intermittent non-erosive arthritis, and Raynaud's phenomenon.

Dry eyes

Symptoms include burning, itching, stinging, tired eyes, photophobia, and occasionally mucus discharge from the eyes. Tear substitutes escalate from watery drops (such as Hypromellose) to more viscous drops. Preservative-free drops are needed if they are used more than six times daily to prevent irritation. Paraffin-based gels help night-time dryness. Severe dry eyes can be helped by permanent or temporarily plugging of the tear duct punctae.

Dry mouth

Symptoms are worsened by some medications such as tricyclic antidepressants, antihistamines, diuretics, and β-blockers, which should be avoided if possible.

Tracheal and nasal dryness means that patients are hypersensitive to atmospheric irritants such as smoking and air-conditioning. Associated symptoms include difficulty in chewing or swallowing, hoarse voice, difficulty in speaking, and swollen salivary glands. Vigilance in checking for dental caries and oral candidiasis is important. Patients are advised to avoid dehydration and seek regular dental care. Fluoride mouthwashes can improve oral hygiene. Salivary substitute sprays with replacement gels give limited symptomatic relief, and in severe cases pilocarpine (muscarinic agonist) in doses increasing from 5mg daily up to 5mg four times daily can help.

Musculoskeletal and systemic features

Musculoskeletal and systemic features are common. Patients may have positive rheumatoid factor and positive ANA. Joints are tender and painful rather than swollen. Some patients present with true inflammatory arthritis, often misdiagnosed as rheumatoid arthritis. Erosive arthritis is very rare. Non-specific systemic features of tiredness, lethargy, malaise, and exhaustion are common. Hydroxychloroquine has been used with anecdotal evidence of effect, particularly helping fatigue and arthralgia.

Interstitial lung disease is seen on high-resolution CT scan in up to 30% of pSS patients in some series. Some present with dry cough or exertion or dyspnoea. The majority are asymptomatic.

Skin rashes and skin dryness

A variety of rashes may occur, including palpable purpura, small-vessel vasculitis, urticaria, and flat purpura. These are often associated with hypergammaglobulinaemia. More than 50% of patients have dry skin resulting from lymphocytic-infiltrated exocrine glands.

Gynaecological and obstetric problems

Vaginal dryness is common and can be helped with over-the-counter vaginal lubricants. Hormone replacement therapy may be appropriated for menopausal patients.

pSS patients have normal fertility. Approximately 1 in 20 pregnancies in Ro-positive individuals are complicated by the development of the neonatal lupus rash. The rash generally appears at approximately 6 weeks of age and fades spontaneously over the subsequent 3 or 4 months. Approximately 30% of mothers have no pSS symptoms at the time of birth, but the majority eventually develop symptoms.

A rarer life-threatening complication is congenital heart block which occurs in <2% of pregnancies with either Ro or La antibodies. Ultrasound scanning from approximately 16 weeks of age can detect this. The risk is increased if a previous child has been born with congenital heart block. It is slightly more common in female children. Seventy-five per cent of affected children survive, but nearly all require pacemakers in the first few months of life.

Thrombocytopenia of the newborn is described, but is a much rarer complication and usually resolves spontaneously.

Neuropsychiatric involvement

Neuropsychiatric involvement is well recognized, with atypical depression, anxiety, and psychosis. Psychological distress with fibromyalgic symptoms are present in >20% of pSS patients. It can be difficult to distinguish fibromyalgia spectrum patients with secondary sicca symptoms from pSS.

4. What are the late complications?

A rare but important late complication of pSS is B-cell lymphoma. Patients often have raised immunoglobulin levels which should be monitored at least annually. B-cell lymphoma affects 1–5% of patients with a relative risk of developing Hodgkin's lymphoma of 44 compared with the normal population. The absolute risk is small and risk factors include the presence of autoantibodies, monoclonal gammopathies, a sudden disappearance of serum immunoglobulins, and disappearance of rheumatoid factor, lymphadenopathy, skin vasculitis, peripheral nerve involvement, low-grade fever, anaemia, major salivary gland swelling, and lymphopenia.

Other comorbidities

Patients commonly have a family history of autoimmune disease. Thyroid disease occurs in ~30% of pSS patients, coeliac disease in up to 15%, and primary biliary cirrhosis in ~5%, and there is an increased association with pernicious anaemia. Other significant comorbidities include depression, fibromyalgic symptoms, and distal renal tubular acidosis.

Further reading

Delalande S, de Seze J, Fauchais A-L, *et al.* (2004). Neurologic manifestations in primary Sjögren syndrome: a study of 82 patients. *Medicine*; **83**: 280–91.

Fox RI, Dixon R, Guarrasi V, Krubel S (1996). Treatment of primary Sjögren's syndrome with hydroxychloroquine: a retrospective, open-label study. *Lupus*; **5**: S31–6.

Kruize AA, Hené RJ, Kallenberg CG, *et al.* (1993). Hydroxychloroquine treatment for primary Sjögren's syndrome: a two year double blind crossover trial. *Ann Rheum Dis*; **52**: 360–4.

Vincent TL, Richardson MP, Mackworth-Young CG, Hawke SH, Venables PJ (2003). Sjögren's syndrome-associated myelopathy: response to immunosuppressive treatment. *Am J Med*; **114**: 145–8.

Vitali C, Bombardieri S, Jonsson R, *et al.* (2002). Classification criteria for Sjögren's syndrome: a revised version of the European criteria proposed by the American–European Consensus Group. *Ann Rheum Dis*; **61**: 554–8.

Case 46

A 22-year-old female marathon runner was attending the sports clinic for management of bilateral insufficiency fractures of the femoral head, confirmed on MRI. This had not occurred in association with any increase in her usual training programme and she was struggling to return to training. She did not have any past medical history of note and was not on any regular medications. On further direct questioning she reported mild proximal weakness in the upper and lower limbs and on examination was noted to have a BMI of 17.2kg/m^2 with normal stature.

Investigations showed the following:

- Hb 10.8g/dL; MCV 72fL
- ALP 320U/L
- Calcium 2.2mmol/L
- PTH 28pg/mL
- 1,25-dihydroxyvitamin D3 7pg/mL
- 25-hydroxyvitamin D3 36ng/mL.

Questions

1. Which underlying causes should be considered and what further information is required to come to a final diagnosis?
2. What is the most likely diagnosis and how should this be treated?
3. What rare diagnosis should be considered if the patient fails to respond to treatment as expected?

Answers

1. Which underlying causes should be considered and what further information is required to come to a final diagnosis?

The low BMI in this female athlete raises the possibility of the female athlete triad. Further corroboration should be sought in the history including evidence of amenorrhoea, poor dietary habits, and laxative and diuretic use. The presence of the female athlete triad increases the risk of osteoporosis, which would be a possible explanation for the development of insufficiency fractures without any increased loading. Other risk factors for osteoporosis should be identified and DEXA scanning should be considered.

Fracture in the context of proximal muscle weakness raises the possibility of osteomalacia, which can be caused by vitamin D deficiency or a PTH-independent defect in renal handling of phosphate. Risk factors for vitamin D deficiency include reduced oral intake, decreased sun exposure, malabsorption, severe liver disease, and renal insufficiency. Ageing is also associated with significantly reduced 1-α-hydroxylase activity in the kidney, and some antiepileptic medications such as phenytoin increase the deactivation of the active metabolite 1,25-dihydroxyvitamin D in the liver.

Characteristic features include bone pain and tenderness, proximal muscle weakness, and non-fragility fracture. In children bone deformity occurs resulting in bowing of weight-bearing bones and irregularity at the metaphyseal–epiphyseal junction which is usually detected at the wrist and costochondral junctions. The latter results in the 'ricketic rosary'. Harrison's groove describes the indentation of the softened ribs at the insertion of the diaphragm. Rapid growth of the softened skull results in frontal bossing and parietal bone flattening. Dentition may also be poor. Laboratory investigations in vitamin D deficiency can show low serum calcium and phosphate, and elevated alkaline phosphatase and PTH.

Vitamin D_2 (ergocalciferol) is obtained from vegetable sources, whereas vitamin D_3 (cholecalciferol) is mainly synthesized in the skin following exposure to UVB light and can also be derived from food sources such as oily fish and fortified foods including milk, juices, and cereals. Both forms of vitamin D are rapidly converted to 25-hydroxyvitamin D in the liver but only a fraction is activated to 1,25-dihydroxyvitamin D by the kidneys. Thus, the former is the best marker of body stores of vitamin D. In vitamin D deficiency 1,25-dihydroxyvitamin D_3 levels may well be normal, whereas low 25-hydroxyvitamin D_3 levels are diagnostic.

Osteomalacia due to altered phosphate homeostasis is rare but gives rise to the same bone histopathology. Causes include the following:

◆ Excess antacid use, often over several years with phosphate-binding antacids.

◆ Idiopathic hypophosphataemia.

◆ X-linked hypophosphataemic rickets which is caused by vitamin D resistance and manifests with short stature and rickets in homozygous males, and variable growth and deformity in females. Early recognition is key in order to prevent long-term deformity.

- Fanconi syndrome is associated with a number of congenital and acquired conditions where proximal renal tubular defects result in glycosuria, aminoaciduria, phosphaturia, and hypophosphataemia.

Laboratory investigations show a very low phosphate and 1,25-dihydroxyvitamin D_3 level with normal or slightly low calcium and normal or slightly elevated PTH. 25-hydroxyvitamin D_3 levels are normal. The biochemical abnormalities detected so far in this case fit with a diagnosis of hypophosphataemic osteomalacia, and serum phosphate levels should be checked.

The presence of a microcytic anaemia also raises the possibility of gastrointestinal malabsorption, which could be associated with coeliac disease. This would account for the low BMI, leading to increased risk of osteoporosis. Malabsorption can also result in vitamin D deficiency and osteomalacia, but the normal 25-hydroxyvitamin D_3 levels make this unlikely unless vitamin D resistance is present.

Further investigations showed:

- serum phosphate 0.48mmol/L
- creatinine 62μmol/L
- urinanalysis normal
- urinary phosphate increased (70mmol/day)
- anti-endomyseal and anti-tissue transglutaminase antibodies normal.

2. What is the most likely diagnosis and how should this be treated?

The most likely diagnosis in this case is idiopathic hypophosphataemic osteomalacia. The treatment depends on the exact underlying cause, but generally includes both phosphate and vitamin D supplementation.

3. What rare diagnosis should be considered if the patient fails to respond to treatment as expected?

If the patient does not respond from a biochemical or clinical perspective, a rare phenomenon to suspect is oncogenic associated osteomalacia. The tumour is usually benign and of mesenchymal origin. The mechanism is not completely elucidated, but it is thought to be mediated by the humoral factor fibroblastic growth factor 23 which deregulates proximal renal tubular phosphate handling. Some improvement can be seen with vitamin D and phosphate supplementation; however, resection of the tumour usually results in cure.

Further reading

Hannan FM, Athanasou NA, Teh J, Gibbons CL, Shine B, Thakker RV (2008). Oncogenic hypophosphataemic osteomalacia: biomarker roles of fibroblast growth factor 23, 1,25-dihydroxyvitamin D3 and lymphatic vessel endothelial hyaluronan receptor 1. *Eur J Endocrinol*; **158**: 265–71.

Kennel KA, Drake MT, Hurley DL (2010). Vitamin D deficiency in adults: when to test and how to treat. *Mayo Clin Proc*; **85**: 752–8.

List of cases by diagnosis
Case 1: Paget's disease
Case 2: Giant cell arteritis
Case 3: Leprosy
Case 4: Sarcoidosis
Case 5: Gout
Case 6: Enteropathic arthritis
Case 7: Haemochromatosis
Case 8: Haemophilia
Case 9: Systemic lupus erythematosus
Case 10: Hypothyroidism
Case 11: Familial Mediterranean fever
Case 12: Marfan's syndrome
Case 13: Antiphospholipid syndrome
Case 14: Osteoporosis
Case 15: Systemic-onset juvenile idiopathic arthritis
Case 16: Ankylosing spondylitis
Case 17: Achilles tendinopathy
Case 18: Adverse neural dynamics
Case 19: HIV
Case 20: Oligoarticular juvenile idiopathic arthritis and uveitis
Case 21: Osteogenesis imperfecta
Case 22: Stress fracture
Case 23: Wegener's granulomatosis
Case 24: Rheumatoid myocarditis
Case 25: Paraneoplastic rheumatic disease
Case 26: CNS vasculitis
Case 27: Complex regional pain syndrome
Case 28: Limited cutaneous systemic sclerosis
Case 29: Antisynthetase syndrome
Case 30: Whipple's disease
Case 31: Female athlete triad
Case 32: Pars defect
Case 33: Anterior knee pain
Case 34: Relapsing polychondritis
Case 35: Eosinophilic fasciitis
Case 36: Rheumatoid vasculitis
Case 37: Septic arthritis
Case 38: Rheumatoid arthritis of the neck
Case 39: Behçet's disease
Case 40: Takayasu's arteritis
Case 41: Raynaud's phenomenon
Case 42: CRMO/SAPHO
Case 43: Viral arthritis
Case 44: Acromegaly
Case 45: Sjögren's syndrome
Case 46: Osteomalacia

List of cases by aetiological mechanisms

Inflammatory arthritis: *16, 24, 36, 37, 38*
Inflammatory autoimmune connective disease: *9, 13, 28, 29, 34, 41, 45*
Other inflammatory conditions: *4, 6, 11, 35, 42*
Paediatric inflammatory conditions: *15, 20*
Vasculitis: *2, 23, 26, 39, 40*
Inherited disorders: *7, 8, 12, 21*
Metabolic: *1, 5, 7, 10, 14, 44*
Soft tissue/sports' injury: *17, 22, 27, 31, 32, 33*
Mechanical dysfunction: *18*
Infection: *3, 19, 37, 43, 30*
Malignancy: *25*

Index

Bold indicates the diagnosis of the case discussed within the page range.

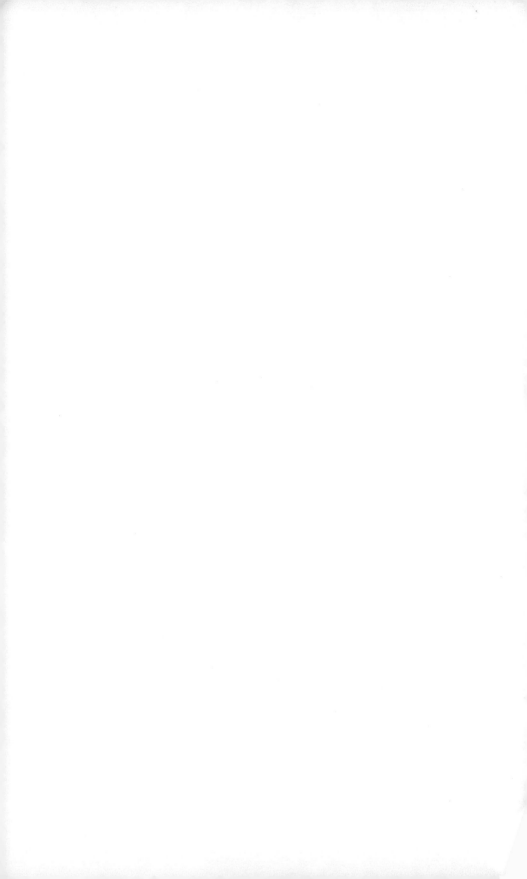